the migraine solution

Trusted Advice for a Healthier Life
from Harvard Medical School

the *migraine* solution

A Complete Guide to Diagnosis, Treatment, and Pain Management

Paul Rizzoli, MD, FAAN,
Elizabeth Loder, MD, MPH,
and Liz Neporent

St. Martin's Griffin New York

www.stmartins.com

Design by Patrice Sheridan

The information in this book is not intended to replace the advice of the reader's own physician or other medical professional. You should consult a medical professional in matters relating to health, especially if you have existing medical conditions, and before starting, stopping, or changing the dose of any medication you are taking. Individual readers are solely responsible for their own health-care decisions. The author and the publisher do not accept responsibility for any adverse effects individuals may claim to experience, whether directly or indirectly, from the information contained in this book.

The fact that an organization or Web site is mentioned in the book as a potential source of information does not mean that the author or the publisher endorses any of the information it may provide or recommendations it may make.

The stories in this book are composite, fictional accounts based on the experiences of many individuals. Similarities to any real person or persons are coincidental and unintentional.

LIBRARY OF CONGRESS CATALOGING-IN-PUBLICATION DATA

Rizzoli, Paul.
The migraine solution : a complete guide to diagnosis, treatment, and pain management / Paul Rizzoli, Elizabeth Loder, Liz Neporent.
p. cm.
ISBN 978-0-312-60581-0 (pbk.)
1. Migraine—Popular works. I. Loder, Elizabeth. II. Neporent, Liz. III. Title.
RC392.R59 2012
616.8'4912—dc23 2011032800

First Edition: January 2012

10 9 8 7 6 5 4 3 2 1

From Elizabeth—To my father, Thomas Wentz

From Paul—To my father, Hugo; my uncle, Lewis; and my aunt, Lilia

From Liz—To my brother Mark and his family

contents

the migraine solution

chapter 1

What Are the Different Types of Headaches?

In the first season of the TV show *Lost,* Sawyer, one of the main characters, experienced headaches. What caused these headaches seemed to be an easily solved mystery: He needed reading glasses, which he managed to find on that mysterious island.

If only all headaches could be cured so quickly. But given the many colorful, bizarre, and even scary names that various types of headaches go by, it's easy to be confused, or even terrified, by this common problem.

There are more than three hundred types of headaches listed in medical books though fewer than 10 percent have a known cause. Medical experts divide headaches into two general categories: *primary* and *secondary.*

Primary headaches aren't the result of any underlying condition or disease; these headaches are self-contained. In other words, once we've arrived at a diagnosis, there's no testing necessary, and we're ready to discuss treatment. Secondary headaches are the symptom of something else, typically a disease, trauma, or brain disorder. If we suspect a secondary cause, you'll need to undergo testing to uncover the principal issue. Of the two, secondary headaches are more worrisome, but this in no way trivializes the pain and suffering someone with a primary headache experiences.

By the way, one frequent concern we often hear from patients is that their head pain moves around. This is actually a good sign. It typically means that there is a benign process at work, and it is almost always a manifestation of a primary headache. It is a reflection that the brain itself, rather than a lesion or an expanding tumor, is causing the problem.

How a Diagnosis Is Made

Making a diagnosis of a primary headache problem like migraines, tension-type, or cluster headaches is not just a matter of ruling out other causes of headache. The International Classification of Headache Disorders (ICHD), which is considered the "bible" for doctors who make headache diagnoses, lists criteria that must be met before a headache diagnosis can be assigned. ICHD classifies headaches based on their predominant characteristics—for example, headaches that are one-sided with typical associated features such as nausea and vomiting generally fit in the "migraine" category. The different headaches may then be broken down into subtypes. Migraines, for instance, can occur with or without aura and can be episodic or chronic. Tension-type headaches can occur with or without muscle tension, and so on.

The ICHD headache categories and criteria were first developed based on the consensus of headache experts—headache is a clinical diagnosis, and there are no tests or X-rays that "prove" someone has a migraine. Instead, the experts identified patterns of symptoms that are common in those with migraines. (This might help you understand why your doctor asks such detailed questions about your headache symptoms when trying to make a diagnosis.)

The ICHD is a work in progress and will undoubtedly be updated periodically in the future although we don't think it's likely the criteria for migraines will change substantially. This is because the original criteria for diagnosing migraines and other disorders, such as cluster headaches, have stood the test of time quite well. Newer imaging techniques that allow us to see which parts of the brain are active during different types of headaches have in large part confirmed earlier expert opinion that these are two separate forms of headache.

Primary Headaches

Tension-type Headaches

Tension-type headaches are the most common type of headache, affecting more than three in four people at some point in their lives. We consider the term itself a misnomer because doctors don't believe that this type of headache is usually caused by muscle tension or stress. As a result, this is a very unsatisfactory and contested diagnosis. Many experts speculate that they are simply a milder form of migraines.

In our practice, we carefully explain the use of the diagnosis because it tends to carry a stigma. Mary came to us having been labeled a tension-headache sufferer several years ago, and one of the first things she told us is how much this bothered her. "It makes me sound like I don't deal well with stress, and I can't get my act together," she said during her initial examination.

As we explained to Mary and tell all patients with a similar syndrome, the diagnosis is not a reflection on how they handle their lives. *Tension-type headache* refers simply to a pattern of headache, a fairly nondescript headache

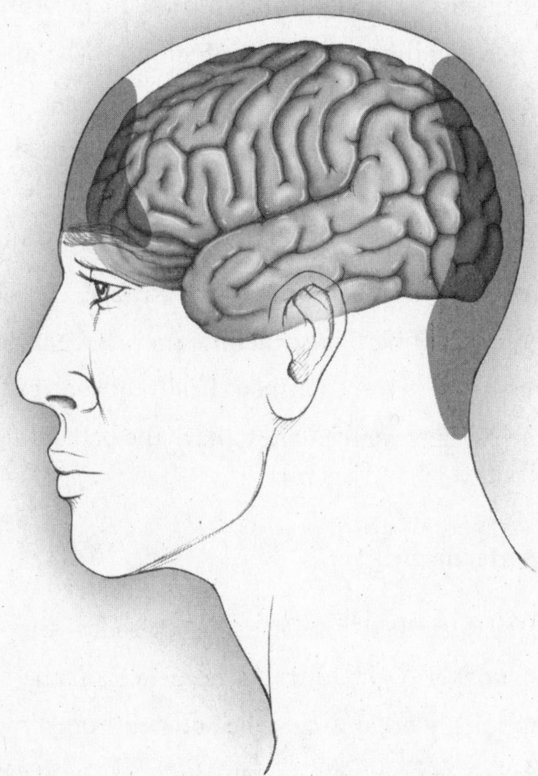

Figure 1: Tension-type headache pain

Tension-type headaches often produce steady pain across the forehead or in the back of the head. Sometimes, the pain is felt throughout the head, and the sensation is often described as a dull tightness.

without many of the classic features of migraines. Unlike migraine headaches, tension-type headaches are not often accompanied by other symptoms, such as nausea, vomiting, or blurred vision. The pain is mild or moderate. It may envelop your entire head or be limited to the forehead or to the back or top of your head. Many people describe the sensation as a dull tightness or pressure that occurs in a bandlike pattern (see Figure 1). The intensity of the pain may fluctuate, but most of the time it won't be severe enough to keep you from functioning or sleeping or to awaken you at night.

Tension-type headaches can occur infrequently, regularly, or daily. They are common at any age, but women are more susceptible: Their lifetime prevalence is 88 percent, versus 68 percent for men. Really, anyone can have one. The patients we see tend to have the bad ones.

Cluster Headaches

When Jay described his headache episodes, they were understandably frightening. As he ticked off the symptoms, it quickly became clear he suffered from a rare but painful class of head pain known as cluster headaches.

Jay's headaches begin suddenly, usually an hour or two after he falls asleep. The pain is intense, sharp, and penetrating, and it usually occurs behind one eye, which can get teary and bloodshot. His eyelid may droop, and the nostril on that side may first be stuffy, then runny. During a single attack, the symptoms can occur in either the left or right side but never in both.

Unlike someone with a migraine headache—who tends to lie quietly in bed—Jay must get up and pace the floor. The pain is so excruciating that it's tempting to bang his head against a wall. After an hour or two, the pain and other symptoms usually recede, sometimes just as suddenly as they came on. But they tend to recur at the same time day after day.

About ten times as many men as women have cluster headaches. About 85 percent of those affected by this type of headache have the episodic form: clusters of one or two headaches a day over a period of two to six weeks, alternating with headache-free stretches. The remission time between cluster periods is generally six to twelve months, but it can be as short as a few weeks or as long as several years. The other 15 percent of those with cluster headaches have the chronic form. In these cases, the attacks continue for at least a year without any remission.

Chronic Daily Headache Syndrome

Suzanne woke up with a headache nearly every day. She started having occasional mild head pain in her twenties, which gradually increased in frequency and intensity and now, in her early thirties, she came to see us for some relief.

Suzanne is among a significant minority of headache sufferers who have frequent headaches. Most people experience headaches only from time to time. But like Suzanne, about one in twenty people experience them daily or almost every day. And women are twice as likely as men to develop chronic daily headache.

Chronic daily headache is a broad term used to describe daily or near-daily headaches that can develop from a number of different causes. In two out of three cases, chronic daily headache develops in people who previously experienced only intermittent migraines, tension headaches, or other types of headaches. If the initial type of headache is known, doctors may use more specific diagnostic terms such as *chronic migraine* or *chronic tension-type headache.* In such people, the headaches tend to increase in frequency gradually—over the course of a decade or so—until they occur daily. In the remaining one-third of cases, chronic daily headache develops without warning, sometimes as a result of illness, surgery, or an injury to the head, neck, or back, and sometimes for no apparent reason.

Regardless of the cause, chronic daily headaches are notoriously difficult to treat and, understandably, often produce anxiety and depression. To make matters worse, about half of people with chronic daily headache syndrome also experience additional and more severe headaches on a regular basis.

Chronic daily headaches usually manifest in one of two distinct patterns. About half of those affected experience headaches that begin in the morning and worsen through the day, while one-quarter experience the reverse (pain that is worst in the morning and gradually diminishes). The remaining one-quarter experience a variable pattern, with pain sometimes diminishing and sometimes worsening as the day goes on.

The types of headaches you've had in the past may also affect symptoms once chronic daily headache develops. Suzanne described her daily headache pain as a steady, viselike grip with throbbing at the temples. Others have a sensory or visual disturbance known as an aura that may or may not diminish in frequency over time. Meanwhile, those with a history of tension-type headaches may sometimes develop nausea and vomiting,

Exploding Head Syndrome

Despite its name, exploding head syndrome isn't actually dangerous; that is, there are no actual head explosions with this condition. A person with exploding head syndrome hears a very loud noise that seems to be coming from inside the head. There's no pain or other physical sensations though the noise can be terribly frightening. Like cluster headaches, exploding head syndrome typically comes on when you're asleep. This is a rare and poorly understood condition and technically is not even a headache disorder. Nonetheless, people with this condition often end up in the headache clinic looking for an explanation. Experts speculate that it may be caused by minor seizures affecting the brain's temporal lobe or a problem in the middle ear. Like so many headaches and other health problems, it seems that stress and fatigue play a role in its onset.

sensitivity to light and noise, and throbbing in the temples—hallmarks of migraines.

Migraine Headaches

Migraine pain has been called indescribable, yet 35 million Americans know it all too well. Twenty-eight million

Americans—about one in five women and one in twenty men—have migraines. We think of a migraine as a "headache plus"; that is, a headache plus a lot of other symptoms. It's a total body syndrome, which horror author Stephen King, himself a migraineur, penned a vivid description of in his novel *Firestarter*:

> The headache would get worse until it was a smashing weight, sending red pain through his head and neck with every pulse beat. Bright lights would make his eyes water helplessly and send darts of agony into the flesh just behind his eyes. Small noises magnified, ordinary noises insupportable. The headache would worsen until it felt as if his head were being crushed inside an inquisitor's lovecap. . . . He would be next to helpless.

Migraine is the French derivation of the Greek word *hemikrania,* meaning "half a head," referring to a typical pattern of migraine distress—pain only on one side of the head, most often at the temple (see Figure 2). The affected side can vary from one attack to the next or during a single episode. One-sided pain is a common but not invariable characteristic of migraines; plenty of sufferers experience bilateral or generalized head pain with migraines.

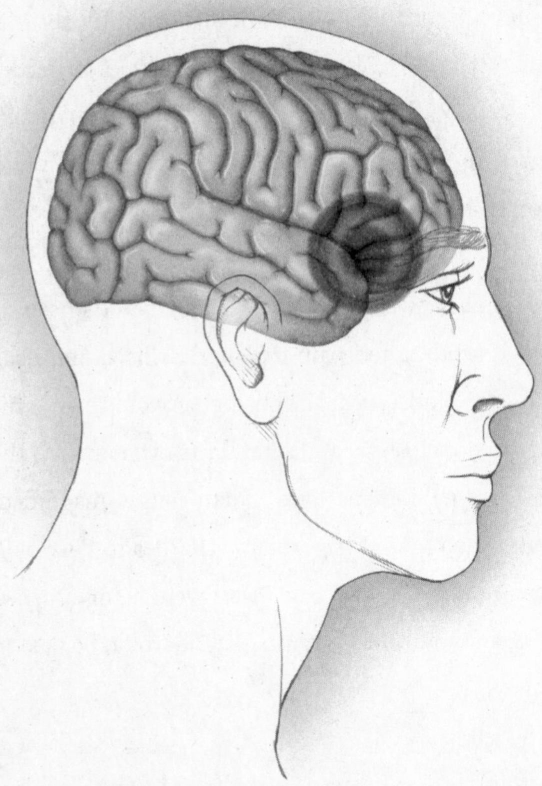

Figure 2: Migraine headache pain
Unlike tension-type and sinus headaches, which produce a dull, steady pain, the pain of migraine headaches is throbbing or sharp. It often occurs only on one side of the head.

Unlike tension-type and sinus headaches, which produce a dull, steady pain, the pain of a migraine headache is throbbing or sharp. It is usually most severely in the area of the temple but may also affect the eye, or back of the head.

The pain ranges from moderate to severe. Unlike tension-type headaches, migraine headaches can keep you from functioning or sleeping, and they can even rouse you from sound slumber. Most people describe the pain as pulsating or throbbing. It can also be sharp, almost as if a dagger is piercing your temple or eye.

Nausea and vomiting are common during a migraine headache. Likewise, tense head, neck, and shoulder muscles can accompany a migraine headache. In most cases, this is thought to be an involuntary response to the pain rather than its cause (although it is probably the case that tight muscles can trigger a migraine headache). Bright lights and loud noises worsen the pain and may prompt someone with a migraine headache to seek out quiet, dimly lit places. Similarly, odors may aggravate nausea and vomiting.

About 20 percent of migraines begin with one or more neurological symptoms called an aura. Visual complaints are most common. They may include halos, sparkles or flashing lights, wavy lines, and even temporary loss of vision. The aura may also produce numbness or tingling on one side of the body, especially the face or hand. Problems with speech can also occur. Some patients develop aura symptoms without getting headaches; they often think they are having a stroke, not a migraine.

The majority of migraines develop without an aura. In typical cases, the pain is on one side of the head, often beginning around the eye and temple before spreading to the back of the head. The pain is frequently severe and is described as throbbing or pulsating. Nausea is common, and many migraine patients have a watering eye, a running nose, or congestion. If these symptoms are prominent, they may lead to a misdiagnosis of cluster or sinus headaches.

Without effective treatment, migraine attacks in adults usually last from four to seventy-two hours. When you're suffering a migraine, even four hours is far too long—and that's why early treatment is so important.

You might also experience a sort of migraine known as aura without headache. This includes many of the symptoms of migraine with aura minus the painful part. For many people, there are clear migraine stages. These include prodrome, with warning signals that a migraine is coming, such as changes in mood or appetite, aura (in about 20 percent of people with migraine), then postdrome, also known as a migraine hangover. Not everyone goes through all the stages—and in the case of aura without headache, the person skips the actual headache.

Secondary Headaches

Secondary headaches are actually symptoms of another health problem. Many non-life-threatening medical conditions, such as a head cold, the flu, or a sinus infection, can cause headache. Some less common but serious causes include bleeding, infection, or a tumor.

A headache can also be the only warning signal of high blood pressure, which your doctor may also refer to as *hypertension.* In addition, certain medications—such as nitroglycerin, prescribed for a heart condition, and estrogen, prescribed for menopausal symptoms—are notorious causes of headaches.

One particularly severe type of secondary headache is called a thunderclap headache. As its name implies, this is a very severe headache that comes on abruptly. It's hard to ignore and feels like someone punched you in the head. In some cases, the headache may start to fade after an hour–but it may last days.

Whether it improves promptly or not, it's important to get immediate medical attention if you suddenly experience

Do you scream after ice cream?

One minute you're enjoying a delicious ice-cream cone; the next, you have "brain freeze." Generally, the headache is immediate and lasts for under a minute. It's usually a very sharp, steady pain felt in the center of the forehead, but it may also occur on one side.

The cause of cold-stimulus headache, stabbing headache, or "ice-cream headache," remains largely a mystery. One theory is that the pain originates in the back of the throat, which is chilled by the ice cream, but is felt in the head—a phenomenon known as referred pain. Any cold food or drink can induce this type of headache, but ice cream is the main culprit because it's very cold and is often swallowed quickly. This doesn't allow for the treat to be warmed slightly in the mouth before it contacts the back of the throat.

To the relief of ice-cream lovers, doctors don't prescribe abstinence for headache prevention. Instead, they suggest taking smaller bites and eating slowly, to give your mouth enough time to warm up the ice cream.

a very severe headache, one you'd describe as "the worst headache of your life." Sudden, severe headaches can be a sign of bleeding in or around the brain, which can be deadly if not treated quickly. Fortunately, thunderclap headaches are not common. However, since it can be hard to tell the difference between dangerous and benign causes of thunderclap headaches, it's prudent to go to a doctor or hospital for evaluation.

How to Think About Your Headaches

Although most people experience at least one headache annually, others suffer from recurring headaches: About 50 percent of people experience a headache at least once a month, 15 percent at least once a week, and 5 percent every day. But only a small fraction of these people ever seek a doctor's attention because most headaches disappear on their own or with the help of an over-the-counter pain reliever, rest, or a good night's sleep. Headaches that are severe, occur often, or are unresponsive to nonprescription pain relievers require medical attention.

When trying to classify your headaches, it helps to step back from each individual headache and think of your entire experience as a syndrome, so you can get a complete picture of your problem. For example, your most recent headache may have been fairly mild even though you endure a real whopper three to four times a year. In our practice we take great care to consider the whole picture to make a diagnosis.

Headaches don't always match their textbook descriptions, and yours may not exactly match any of the descriptions in this chapter. Often, the symptoms of different types of headaches can occur in conjunction. Many people suffer from a hybrid of tension and migraine headaches, which can cause confusion because there isn't a definitive test for either type of headache. A headache produced by stress or tight muscles can also resemble one caused by an underlying disease. To exclude more serious causes, when indicated, your doctor may perform additional tests, possibly including a computed tomography (CT) scan or a magnetic resonance imaging (MRI) scan of your head or neck.

It's also important to keep in mind that your pain patterns may not exactly fit any of the descriptions above—but it's a pretty safe bet that you have your own stereotypical and instantly recognizable pattern. In other words, you can always sense when your headache is coming on, and you have a pretty good idea of how it will play out. You can take care of many types of headaches by yourself, and your doctor can give you medication to control most of the tougher ones. But some headaches call for prompt medical care. You should know when a headache needs urgent care (see box on page 20) and how to control the vast majority of headaches that are not threatening to your health.

Doctors don't fully understand what causes most headaches. They do know that the brain tissue itself and the bones of the skull are never responsible since they don't have nerves that register pain. But the blood vessels in the head and neck can signal pain, as can the tissues that surround the brain and some major nerves that originate in the brain. The scalp, sinuses, teeth, and muscles and joints of the neck can also cause head pain. For most of us, an occasional headache is nothing more than a temporary speed bump in the course of a busy day. But for some of us, headaches are a big problem.

Although headaches are rarely harbingers of more ominous disease, it makes sense to see your doctor if you're having a headache on a weekly basis, if your headaches interfere with your ability to function, or if they change in any particular way. Most likely, your headaches aren't a symptom of anything serious, but the peace of mind and possibility of effective treatment justify the time and expense of a medical evaluation. In the case of migraines, it's more than just peace of mind. You deserve to be appropriately diagnosed and treated.

When to Worry

You can take care of many types of headaches by yourself, and your doctor can give you medication to control most of the tougher ones. But some headaches call for prompt medical care. Here are some warning signs:

- Headaches that first develop after age fifty
- A major change in the pattern of your headaches
- An unusually severe "worst headache ever"
- Pain that increases with coughing or movement
- Headaches that get steadily worse
- Changes in personality or mental function
- Headaches that are accompanied by fever, stiff neck, confusion, decreased alertness or memory, or neurological symptoms such as visual disturbances, slurred speech, weakness, numbness, or seizures
- Headaches that are accompanied by a painful red eye
- Headaches that are accompanied by pain and tenderness near the temples in older individuals
- Headaches after a blow to the head
- Headaches that prevent normal daily activities
- Headaches that come on abruptly, especially if they wake you up
- Headaches in patients with cancer or impaired immune systems

chapter 2

What Is a Migraine?

At about two o'clock in the afternoon, Pavi got that familiar feeling. It started with sparkling flashes that seemed to lurk just behind her vision, followed soon after by an upset stomach and a darkening mood. As the pressure gradually increased over her left eye, she knew a crushing headache was on its way.

When Pavi first became a patient, she reported at least eight similar episodes a month—two a week—and the frequency had been gradually escalating for about a decade. After doing a physical exam and taking a complete medical history that included reviewing her headache and medication log (see chapter 4), it was quickly apparent to us that Pavi suffers from migraines.

Though certainly not everyone experiences a migraine the same way or even the same way every time, Pavi's description of the onset of a migraine attack is fairly typical. And if you have severe headaches like this, then you understand that a migraine is more than just a particular type of head pain—it is a broader set of changes that can occur throughout the body although not all of the symptoms are evident in every person who has migraines.

Prodrome and Auras

Some people use the term *migraine* to describe any relentless headache, but not all severe headaches are migraines nor are all migraines severe, although many do live up to their reputation for excruciating pain. Typically, the early sensations that Pavi describes are known as prodromal symptoms or the prodrome, and they warn that a migraine headache is about to commence.

Some migraines are preceded by an aura. The word *aura* isn't just used by psychics. It's also the word used to describe the visual, language, or sensory disturbances some people experience before they get a migraine. These might include seeing things such as halos, bursts of lights or flashing zigzag lines (scintillations). These are often referred to as "positive aura symptoms" since they involve seeing something. There are also "negative aura symptoms" which involve a *loss* of vision, either partially or completely. Most auras include a mixture of these positive and negative symptoms and often change over time. For example, a small area of visual loss (a blind spot) may enlarge or appear to move within the timespan of an episode. A migraine that begins with an aura was once called a classic migraine as opposed to a common migraine, which is not preceded by an aura. Though you may still hear these terms used, we consider them outdated.

A typical visual migraine aura is often characterized by a blind spot or area in one side of the field of vision, known as a scotoma. Often shaped like a thick crescent, the scotoma typically appears as a shimmering zigzag that moves across one side of a person's field of vision, from just off the center, as represented in Figure 3. This phenomenon lasts between twenty minutes and an hour and is often but not always followed by headache and the other typical features of a migraine. In Pavi's case, it's a sparkling sensation she refers to as a *ghost headache* because it often portends the pain to come.

About 20 percent of people with migraines often or always experience headaches that begin with one or more neurological symptoms that can be classified as an aura.

Visual complaints are most common though not all visual disturbances qualify as an aura. For example, some people report blurred vision, but since aura symptoms must be true focal neurological events, this does not qualify as such. Though this may seem like a minor point, it's actually an important distinction since a diagnosis of aura for young women in particular means they should be cautious about using birth-control methods containing estrogen.

Less often, people will experience tingling on one side of the body, often in the hand, arm, or face. Some people experiencing an aura for the first time are sure they are having a stroke. The symptoms of both conditions overlap, but there are distinctions. Auras very often include the flashes of light and the visual hallucinations such as the crescents described above as well as areas of diminished or absent vision or blind spots; the onset and cessation of these symptoms is gradual. In contrast, the symptoms of strokes and other related health issues usually come on suddenly and mainly include the negative symptoms mentioned earlier, such as loss of vision, sensation or movement. So we recommend getting a medical evaluation if you aren't sure what's going on, especially if you don't have a history of migraines.

The majority of migraines develop without an aura. The migraine headache, with or without an aura, tends to produce pain that usually begins (and sometimes stays) on one side of the head. Many people also experience nausea, extreme sensitivity to light or sound, or both. But, as with an aura, you need to be careful about generalizing: Some studies have found that about 40 percent of migraineurs have headache pain on both sides of the head, not just one, and children with migraines usually have pain on both sides; some people experience a shifting of pain from one side to the other during an episode. One way to remember the features of migraines is to use the acronym *POUND* (P is for pulsating pain; O for one-day duration of severe untreated attacks; U for unilateral (one-sided) pain; N for nausea and vomiting; D for disabling intensity).

Many migraine attacks occur on the weekends, in the evening, or at night and, ironically, may be the result of the body's attempt to relax after the day's stresses since for unclear reasons, relaxation sometimes seems to lower an individual's headache threshold, particularly when it comes after a prolonged period of stress. Thus, an evening or nighttime migraine may be more prone to occur after a particularly intense day or a period of prolonged stress.

Both the frequency and the duration of migraine headaches vary from person to person. Without effective treatment, migraine headaches usually last four to seventy-two

Migraine with Aura—The Typical and the Not-So-Typical

Imagine you are speaking when all of a sudden everything that comes out of your mouth is complete gibberish. Your eye begins twitching, and when you look at a book, part of the page looks blank. Many of your symptoms mimic a stroke, but when you rush to the doctor, these symptoms are fading and have been replaced by a bad headache. Instead of seeming worried, they tell you you most likely have a condition known as migraine aura. You may also hear this condition referred to in the media as a *complex migraine*, but this is not the term most medical professionals will use in reference to it.

Aura symptoms and signs do sometimes mimic those of a stroke, but unlike a stroke, the blood flow to your brain is not permanently disrupted, and neurological symptoms—though confusing and scary—are almost always temporary. One reason aura is often misdiagnosed is because it isn't always accompanied by a headache or the migraine headache that follows doesn't develop until later. In other cases, the symptoms may last longer than the hour or so that is typical for most auras. That happens occasionally, and it is worth remembering that there is nothing magic about the figure of an hour that is usually given as the length beyond which an aura should not persist. As long as the symptoms are otherwise typical of an aura, and especially in cases where the person has other similar auras that last no more than an hour, the most likely diagnosis remains aura.

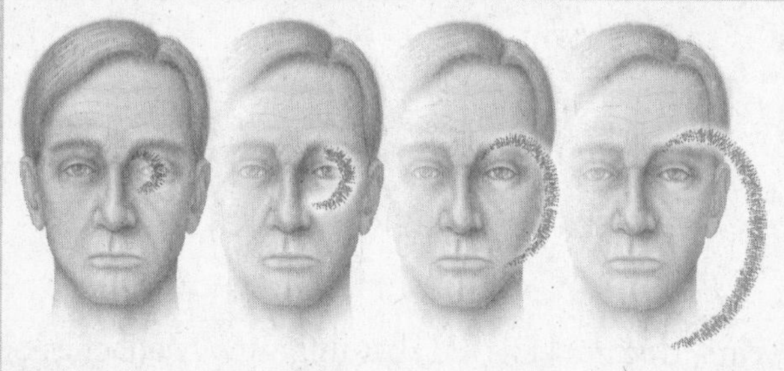

Figure 3: The visual aura of a migraine: scintillating scotoma

Like all migraines, migraines occurring with auras are more commonly suffered by women but can affect anyone at any age. If you experience any of the symptoms described above, or more alarming symptoms, such as a loss of sensation or muscle weakness, you should seek evaluation and treatment, particularly if symptoms persist beyond an hour or so.

hours in adults. And, on occasion, they can persist for days, especially in women who have these headaches before or during menstruation. When a single migraine lasts longer than seventy-two hours it is known as status migrainosus. However long a migraine lasts, we know from the people we see in our practice that, when you're suffering a migraine, even a few hours is far too long—and that's why early treatment is so important.

What Causes a Migraine?

For years, doctors believed that migraine headaches originated with the blood vessels, particularly those that supply the meninges, the thin membranes wrapped around the brain inside the skull. It was thought that when those blood vessels widened—dilated is the medical term—they impinged on pain receptors on the lacy network of trigeminal nerves that service the meninges and other parts of the head. According to this vascular theory, aura was caused by low blood supply from the narrowing of those blood vessels before they rebounded and widened, causing pain. The vascular explanation had considerable intuitive appeal because of the pulsating quality of migraine headaches. Some doctors elaborated on the theory, assigning different sorts of pain to different blood vessels.

But now there is near-total agreement that migraines originate in the brain, not with the blood vessels that surround it. One prevailing theory is that migraine auras are caused by orderly waves of brain-cell activity crossing the cortex, the thin outer layer of brain tissue, followed by periods of decreased activity. The unwieldy (and potentially confusing) name for this phenomenon is cortical spreading depression. A Brazilian researcher, Aristides Leão, first observed it in rat brains in 1944, but many studies support the theory that it occurs in the human brain as well.

Cortical spreading depression makes sense as a cause of aura, but researchers have also linked it to headache. Proponents cite experimental evidence that suggests it sets off inflammatory changes around blood vessels and other processes that stimulate pain receptors from the trigeminal nerves. This "neurogenic" inflammation and the release of other factors make the receptors—and the parts of the brain that receive their signals—increasingly sensitive, so migraines become more likely.

Some leading researchers have expressed doubt about whether all migraines start with cortical spreading depression or just those in which an aura occurs. Experimental drugs that inhibit cortical spreading depression have been developed, but study results reported in 2009 for one of the most promising, a drug called tonabersat, showed a preventive effect on auras, but not on migraine headaches.

So, say some researchers, migraines are best explained as beginning lower in the brain, in the brain stem. This "primitive" region of the brain controls basic functions, such as respiration and responses to pain, and modulates many others, including incoming sensory information. The theory is that if certain areas of the brain stem aren't working properly or are easily excited, they're capable of starting cascades of neurological events, including cortical spreading depression, that account for a migraine's multiple symptoms.

At this point, there are no blood tests for migraines. MRI and CT scans can show brain or other abnormalities that may account for some headaches, such as an aneurysm or brain tumor, but, in general, MRIs and CT scans are normal in migraineurs. MRIs in patients with migraines with an aura sometimes show tiny bright white spots known as white-matter lesions. The cause and consequences of these are not yet known although there is growing evidence they may be a reflection of either vascular or metabolic problems in the brain. Right now, a finding of these typical white-matter changes on an MRI in someone who has migraines with an aura is not considered a cause for alarm; nor does it alter treatment for the headaches. Nonetheless, it is helpful to understand the genesis of your headaches so that these changes will not be misinterpreted as owing to something else. Because proper diagnosis of headaches and treatment can help improve your headache problem, it is important to remember that in many cases, special testing is not necessary to make a diagnosis.

Who Gets Migraines?

It's well documented that women are about three times more likely to have migraines than men, that the tendency to have migraines runs in families, and that they occur less often as people age. During childhood, migraines affect boys and girls equally. But after puberty, the situation shifts, with women more likely to experience migraine headaches. That said, it's still common for men to experience them.

About 9 percent of men and 16 percent of women suffer from migraines each year; the percentage of people who suffer from a migraine at some point during their life is much higher. There also seems to be a connection with motion sickness: Many adult migraine sufferers recall bouts of car sickness as children. But, obviously, these are guideposts, not diagnostic criteria. So, in short, arriving at a definition and diagnosis for migraines is complicated.

Migraines and Stomach Upset

During a migraine headache, arteries in the head dilate. The widened arteries stimulate nerve fibers that encircle the arteries, causing them to send impulses to the brain. There, these nerve impulses are interpreted as pain. They also activate the autonomic nervous system (ANS), which originates in the spinal cord and extends to organs throughout the body, including the stomach and intestines. The ANS controls the body's "fight or flight" response, mobilizing the body for action by speeding up the heart rate, raising blood pressure, and slowing digestion. To slow digestion, the ANS closes the pyloric sphincter (the ring of smooth muscle that separates the stomach from the upper part of the intestines). As a result, the stomach dilates, and any leftover food stays in the stomach, which can cause the nausea and vomiting that often accompany migraine headaches. (There's also evidence that activation of the vomiting centers of the brain occurs as well.) This phenomenon also explains why migraine medications taken by mouth aren't effective for everyone—they aren't always well absorbed into the bloodstream.

chapter 3

Migraine Triggers

Just as Superman has his Kryptonite, every migraineur seems to have a headache trigger. For Katie, it's red wine, especially if she hasn't had a lot of sleep. Even a few sips after a night of tossing and turning virtually guarantees a pounding headache and upset stomach. David thinks that stress is his downfall, though oddly, he's noticed the migraines come a while after the tense moments have passed. And Christina swears that whenever she eats anything with soy in it, she gets a headache within the hour.

A trigger is anything that sets off a migraine. This is different from what we in our practice refer to as an activating factor such as a head injury, puberty, or genetics—anything that starts the ball rolling on headaches and makes a person more susceptible to them in the first place. It's also different from risk factors, such age, sex, or education, attributes that increase your chances of having migraines or having increasingly severe migraines. In contrast, a trigger is the thing (or things) that prompts an individual episode.

Although a migraine can come on without warning, it is often set off by a trigger. Triggers certainly vary from person to person, but a migraine sufferer usually remains sensitive to the same triggers over and over again. It may seem like you become more or less susceptible to your triggers over time, but we suspect you are more likely experiencing a change in headache threshold. Although there is very little research to back this up, we have found that as headaches become more frequent and escalate in intensity, they are triggered more easily; something you were previously able to tolerate may now push you over the edge.

How does a trigger spur a migraine headache? Experts don't know for sure whether it first causes dilation or inflammation of blood vessels or whether some triggers activate brain mechanisms that provoke headaches. There are staunch partisans for each view. Indeed, different triggers may work through different mechanisms. Many of these things are interconnected, and their interaction may foster a migraine headache once it's started.

For instance, inflammation that occurs during a migraine attack can cause widening of blood vessels in the thin meningeal tissues that surround the brain and spinal cord and may make adjacent nerves much more sensitive to signals that ordinarily they ignore. To further complicate matters, researchers believe that different triggers affect these things in different ways.

Many migraine sufferers report sensitivity to strong sensory inputs such as bright lights, loud noises, and smells. Some find it difficult to tolerate ordinary levels of these things, which makes the events of everyday life—such as sitting next to a man wearing too much aftershave—very challenging. But, really, the list of triggers is too long and diverse to cover every single trigger that's ever reported, even in our single practice. What follows is a list of some of the triggers most commonly reported in studies of migraine patients.

Food

For some migraine sufferers, alcohol or a particular food may prompt an attack (see "Migraine Menu"). The list is long, but foods most commonly associated with headache include chocolate and aged cheeses; as well as additives like nitrates, found in most cured meats; and monosodium glutamate (MSG), an ingredient in some canned, processed, and Chinese foods.

Although food and alcohol are often cited by patients as headache triggers, not all common food triggers will set off a migraine in any one individual. Therefore, migraineurs need not avoid all the potential triggers if there is clearly no relationship between their headaches and those substances. Furthermore, there is little good information about how long it takes for most suspected food triggers to cause headaches, and the timing must depend a great deal upon the individual substance, making it difficult to pinpoint the offending food. Although data regarding the role of food in triggering headaches is controversial, we believe that some migraineurs may indeed be susceptible to certain foods as potential triggers, and often these individuals have already identified such triggers themselves by the time they first meet with us.

Chocolate is one food in particular where the evidence is confusing. Many people, especially women, believe that chocolate sets off a migraine, but research is contradictory. In fact, it is possible that a craving for chocolate is an early sign of the beginning of a migraine rather than a cause. So even though it may be useful to track how food affects your headaches, you do need to be careful about jumping to conclusions about how the two things are linked.

Our overarching view on food as a migraine trigger is that if someone is doing well on medication, then following a strict "migraine avoidance diet" might be more trouble than it's worth. However, we've included some commonly mentioned food triggers in the Migraine Menu because so many people feel it can be empowering to take control of something that's related to their headaches, especially when they first try to get a handle on them. We counsel patients who are interested in dietary triggers of headaches to watch for associations between what they eat and how they feel but not to get so caught up in the process that they make themselves crazy.

And, of course, if you suspect a certain food is a trigger, your prevention strategy is simple: Avoid it. Migraine diets like the one we include here are still widely available and are still recommended by certain practitioners and in lay publications on headache. But once again, headache clinics like ours often recognize that for many patients, the considerable effort involved to start and maintain one of these diets is not worth the typically meager results. Furthermore, good-quality research studies often fail to back up specific claims of benefit from these diets. One study suggested that headache improvement might result from any sort of supervised diet, perhaps because when following a diet people are careful to eat on time and avoid the headache trigger of missed meals. It is also possible that expectations of improvement play a role in headache reduction.

Specific dietary triggers aside, the importance of eating regularly cannot be overemphasized, as skipping meals can trigger headaches. Skipped meals and fasting are reported by more than half of migraine sufferers as a trigger in population-based studies. Researchers believe the mechanism could be an alteration in brain chemicals or hormones or a shift in metabolic processes. It is unlikely that the cause is hypoglycemia since blood glucose levels in most people are tightly regulated by the body. In many cases, going as little as five hours without food was enough to bring on a pounding headache in some people.

Alcohol

What doesn't seem to be controversial is the role of alcohol as an important headache trigger for some people with migraines. Just ask Katie. A few sips of wine—especially when she's tired—and she can't function for nearly an entire day. She doesn't drink anymore. It isn't worth it.

Migraine Menu

If you think the effort is worth it, a food diary may help you discover whether something you eat or drink could be provoking your headaches. Foods and additives that sometimes have been named as triggers for a migraine headache include:

- alcoholic beverages
- avocados
- bananas
- beans (except green or wax)
- caffeinated beverages (tea, coffee, cola, etc.)
- cheeses, aged and unpasteurized (Brie, Camembert, Cheddar, Gruyère, Stilton, etc.)
- chicken livers
- chocolate
- citrus fruits
- fermented, pickled, or marinated foods
- herring
- monosodium glutamate (MSG)
- nitrates (found in cured meats)
- nuts and peanut butter
- onions

(cont'd)

- peas
- pork
- sour cream
- vinegar (except white)
- yogurt

Alcohol can have an immediate (within three hours) or delayed "hangover" effect. Some patients have even told us that it can trigger a headache within minutes. But whether red wine is more likely than white wine to induce a migraine is still a matter of discussion; most wine contains chemicals such as sulfites and flavonoids, which can theoretically precipitate migraines.

For those susceptible to migraines, getting a headache does not necessarily depend on how much they drink, and in fact may be more common in light or moderate drinkers than regular heavy drinkers, possibly because heavy drinkers might not drink in the first place if alcohol was a trigger. Though the cause of an immediate alcohol-triggered headache is probably somehow related to dilation of blood vessels in the head, the exact cause of a hangover headache is unknown. It may be due to alteration of sleep patterns, some type of inflammation, or even depletion of magnesium or other indirect effects. Patients who are prone to alcohol-induced migraines should drink in moderation and stay well hydrated, or, like Katie, steer clear of alcohol altogether if possible.

Caffeine

For migraine sufferers, caffeine is both good and bad news. The good news is that some people find that simply drinking a caffeinated beverage can ease their migraine headache. This is because caffeine has some mild pain-relieving properties in its own right, may constrict blood vessels, and also increases the absorption of other pain medications that might be taken with it, such as aspirin or acetaminophen. This is why certain headache-relief drugs such as Cafergot®, Fiorinal®, and Excedrin® contain caffeine and why many people with migraines find that starting the day with a coffee or even a cola drink will keep their headaches at bay.

Now for the bad news: Once the stimulating effects of caffeine wear off, you can crash hard, especially if you haven't had anything to eat. And, as a diuretic, caffeine may dehydrate you. Regular use of fairly ordinary amounts of caffeine, particularly in women, has also been associated with an increased likelihood of the headache worsening over time though the reason for this is not clear.

Excessive use of caffeine-containing headache or pain medicines is associated with medication-overuse headaches, commonly called "rebound" headaches. We've seen in our practice many patients who have unintentionally made their headache problem much worse after taking more and more over-the-counter remedies in response to having headaches; they find themselves in an endless loop of headache and medication, not realizing that the cure is actually part of their problem. Often, people don't see over-the-counter pills as a danger because they don't require a prescription. In addition to escalating headaches, however, drugs that contain aspirin or its relatives or acetaminophen can also create a host of other health issues, such as ulcers and liver problems. If you find yourself taking them on a regular basis, you need to consult with a doctor.

Headaches also occur with abrupt withdrawal or a sudden decrease of caffeine, usually in people who regularly consume at least 200 mg daily, the amount found in about two cups of brewed coffee. One clue to caffeine-withdrawal headaches is that they are especially likely to occur in the morning since overnight is the longest period of time many people will go without ingesting caffeine of any sort. The higher the level of baseline caffeine use, the greater the likelihood of a withdrawal headache,

Caffeine Content	
All figures are approximate, especially with coffee. Different varieties have different caffeine content, and the way the coffee is roasted or prepared can also change the values.	
Double espresso (2 oz.)	45–100 mg
Brewed coffee (8 oz.)	60–120 mg
Instant coffee (8 oz.)	70 mg
Decaf coffee (8 oz.)	1–5 mg
Tea—black (8 oz.)	45 mg
Tea—green (8 oz.)	20 mg
Tea—white (8 oz.)	15 mg
Coca-Cola (12 oz. can)	34 mg
Pepsi (12 oz. can)	38 mg
Root beer (12 oz. can)	22 mg
Noncola beverage (12 oz.)	0 mg
Chocolate milk (8 oz.)	4 mg
Dark chocolate (1 oz.)	20 mg
Milk chocolate (1 oz.)	6 mg
Coffee fudge frozen yogurt (8 oz.)	85 mg

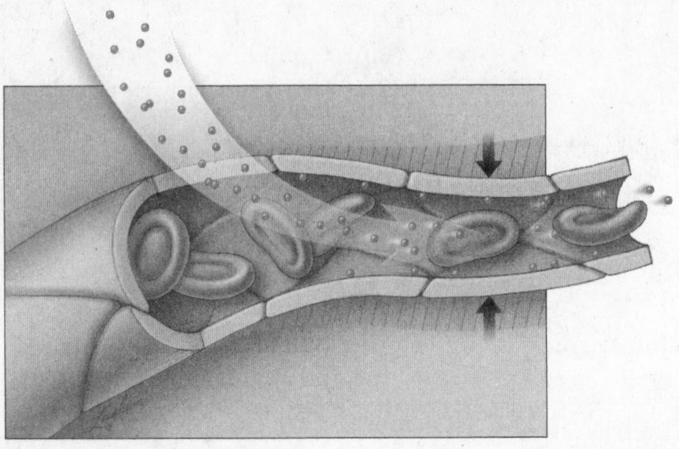

Figure 4: Weekend Woes
Migraine headaches may be more common on weekends, perhaps because many people drink less coffee on weekends or have their first cup later than usual.

although headaches can occur even when patients consuming 100 mg daily stop abruptly. Migraine-susceptible patients should consider limiting their daily intake to less than 200 mg of caffeine a day, realizing that caffeine also is found in tea, cola, chocolate, and even some noncola beverages so you need to be sure to read labels. If you take caffeine-containing medications, limit them to two days a week and check in with your doctor about using them wisely. If you decide to step down your caffeine intake, do it gradually over a period of weeks to avoid having a whopper of a withdrawal headache.

Sleep

Lack of sleep can be a trigger, but so can sleeping too much; waking up from a sound sleep, particularly in the early morning hours, is a well-known migraine symptom. Sleep deprivation may lead to changes in the levels of key proteins that affect nerves involved in pain transmission. In particular, those who experience a deprivation of REM sleep, the stage of sleep characterized by rapid eye movements and dreaming, seem to struggle with migraines the most. This seems to support previously mentioned clinical data associating quality of sleep and migraines.

Sleep and migraines may have a chicken-and-egg connection, at least in children. Another 2010 study, this time performed at St. Christopher's Hospital for Children in Philadelphia, linked kids' migraines to sleep issues. The study found that children with migraines were twice as likely as children with other types of headaches to have sleep apnea, otherwise known as sleep-disordered breathing, which involves repeated arousals from sleep because the upper airway for breathing has been obstructed. Severe migraines were also associated with shorter total sleep time, longer total time to fall asleep, and shorter REM sleep. This is good information for parents of little migraineurs to be aware of, as lack of sleep can have an impact on school, friends, and other aspects of a child's life.

Another study showed an association between poor sleep in adults and all types of headaches, particularly migraines. In this study, older obese men who snored and suffered from sleep apnea had a greater risk of experiencing headache pain than other groups.

Hormones

Most headache triggers affect both men and women. However, there's little doubt that women are more susceptible to migraines in general, and it is likely that this is related to the effects of female hormones on the brain. Many women with migraines report they are more susceptible to headaches in the days just before and after menstrual bleeding begins. Good evidence suggests that the drop in estrogen levels that occurs at this time makes headaches especially likely to occur. Estrogen has long been linked to headaches. A drop in estrogen levels after childbirth or during the placebo-pill week of the birth-control pill may also make headaches more likely to occur in women who are already prone to them.

Migraine headaches that occur around menstruation are reported by some women to be particularly severe and incapacitating. Research suggests that estrogen affects pain pathways by influencing levels or effects of brain chemicals (neurotransmitters). Estrogen also may have a direct effect on blood vessels. Once menopause is well established, many women whose headaches have previously been linked with hormonal changes report headache improvement, but this is not always the case. In some individuals, they may even worsen, and, occasionally, migraines can even start at this point. Even after menopause, women have more migraines than men.

Birth-control pills that contain both estrogen and progestins (combination pills) are suspected of increasing the frequency or intensity of attacks in some patients and in general should be used with caution in those whose migraines are preceded by an aura because of safety concerns. In many women with migraines, though, the birth-control pill (or any hormone containing a birth-control delivery system such as the patch) may have little or no effect on headaches and can be used without worsening of headaches, contrary to some recommendations that use of estrogen-containing contraceptives should be avoided by any woman who suffers from migraines. There is no good way to predict which women with migraines will experience more severe headaches on the pill. If you are worried about this possibility, progesterone-only birth-control methods are not suspected of aggravating migraines, and can be safely used by women who have auras. They are, however, not quite as effective in preventing pregnancy, and they tend to have a few more side effects than combination pills.

The traditional way of giving combination birth-control pills involved taking active, hormone-containing pills for three weeks, then taking a week of placebo (inactive) pills. The lack of hormones during that week caused shedding of the uterine lining (withdrawal bleeding); this was thought to be desirable because it reassured women they were not pregnant. There is some evidence that continuous or extended-duration use of birth-control pills (skipping the placebo [inactive] pills) may lessen the severity of menstrual migraine since estrogen levels do not decline. Most experts feel this continuous use is probably no more risky than the use of the monthly cycling pill since there is no medical or health reason that withdrawal bleeding needs to occur on a monthly basis.

In truth, it's unclear whether or not hormone-containing birth control plays a role in migraines or not. Some of our female patients tell us they seem to while others tell us they don't. It's a tough question to answer because women often start on birth control right around the age they also commonly begin having migraines. In addition to being a potential trigger, could they also be an activating factor? It's hard to say. Researchers and practitioners are still trying to sort this issue out. In the meantime, it is important to remember that while headaches are something women wish to avoid, unwanted pregnancy is also a serious problem, and the combination pill is the most effective form of birth control. These things must be factored into each woman's decision about what is right for her. We discuss all of the aspects related to women and migraines at great length in chapter 7.

Stress as a Trigger

One of the most commonly mentioned migraine triggers, emotional stress, is also one of the most poorly understood. For most patients, the last thing they want to hear in the midst of a bad migraine is a suggestion that the pounding pain spreading across their left eyebrow is the direct result of a bad day at the office.

When reviewing a patient history, we take into account that there are two types of stress that can be a factor in migraines: daily-grind stress, which includes everyday events like traffic jams, screaming babies, and arguing with a spouse, and big-ticket stress such as marriage, divorce, and a death in the family. In general, we have found that the daily-grind stress probably has the biggest effect on migraine frequency. For example, one large study of adolescents found those who had endured long periods of physical and mental abuse were more likely than average to experience chronic daily headaches. Also, a large study found that those who feel they have a lot of stress in their lives, whether they are sweating the small stuff or the big stuff, typically have a higher incidence of headaches than those who aren't as stressed-out. Interestingly, as our patient David seems to find, migraines tend to start not during moments of great stress but later on, as we wind down. We're not clear why this might be—perhaps it is related to changes in levels of the stress hormone cortisol—but many of our patients confirm that this is the case, and the phenomenon is so well recognized that it is often termed *let-down headache*.

Weight Gain

There is no evidence that high body weight or high body mass index (BMI)—which is a measure of body fat based on your height and weight—causes migraines to begin in the first place. However, if you are already plagued by migraines, there is evidence from the Frequent Headache Epidemiology Study that those who are overweight or obese are more likely to experience worsening headaches over time. Since adipose, or fat, tissue is metabolically active and contains inflammatory substances, and inflammation is thought to play a role in migraines, that makes a certain amount of sense. To date, no one has done the study that would be the next step—showing that losing weight improves headaches—but we think the matter deserves attention. There are many other good reasons to maintain a normal body weight, so we do counsel our patients to exercise, eat right, and strategize with them about how to achieve a normal weight. Many of our patients have reported these things help to improve their headaches over the long run.

Trigger Loading

Katie, you'll remember, suspected that red wine was a particularly potent trigger when she lacked sleep. It's possible she's onto something. Many triggers are probably, by themselves, quite weak, but when added together may be sufficient to cause a headache, a concept known as trigger loading. In other words, one trigger in and of itself might not be potent enough to initiate a headache, but when combined, triggers become powerful enough to tip you over the edge.

Migraineurs may have identified dozens of triggers, and it's often impossible to avoid all of them. What's more, the effect of given triggers on your headache can be unpredictable, especially how they may interact with one another. For example, stress might not cause an attack without associated fatigue. And as Katie found, she can sometimes get away with a little wine if she's had a good night's rest.

Summing It All Up

We hope this chapter enlightened you about what triggers are and gave you some clues so you have an idea where to start looking. But even armed with this information, we encourage you to start with a blank slate. The bottom line is that each migraine sufferer is unique, and susceptibility to triggers varies.

Common Triggers

People with migraine headaches cited the following as the top five headache triggers:

- stress or tension
- missing meals
- fatigue
- lack of sleep
- smoke or some sort of odor

chapter 4

Evaluating and Tracking Your Migraines

During her initial appointment, Leslie told us that when she first began having headaches, she tried to shrug them off. She believed the pain was "all in her head," a totally psychological phenomenon and since it wasn't like her leg was broken or she had a perpetual stomachache, it was difficult for her to reconcile herself to the fact that migraines are, indeed, a real medical problem. Like many migraine sufferers, she'd tried to deal with her headaches on her own for quite some time with over-the-counter medications, coffee, or by simply ignoring them when she could. She's at the point now where the suffering interferes with her life so often, she finally decided to seek medical attention.

One of Leslie's biggest concerns is that her headaches are a symptom of something more serious. Could she have a brain tumor? Are her headaches a symptom of some terrible disease or infection? She admits this worry is what finally drove her to pick up the phone and make an appointment.

Once you make the decision to take control of your headaches, you, too, will probably decide to see a doctor. In order to make the most of your visit, we suggest you gather important information that will give your doctor the clues needed to help you with your problem and get to the heart of the matter.

Headache Journal

During the initial consultation, Leslie presented us with a thoroughly detailed headache and medication log using the template on pages 56–57. She had faithfully charted the course of her migraines, noting the intensity, when each had started, and how long it had lasted. She had dutifully checked off the symptoms for each occurrence as well as the steps she had taken to alleviate the attack.

A headache diary can be valuable in helping you and your doctor diagnose and treat your headaches. It can help in identifying possible triggers and related symptoms, as well as tracking the dosage and effectiveness of any medications you're taking.

You can use a preprinted form or a regular calendar or notebook to record this information. There are even "apps" available for your smartphone that can help you track your headaches. Your doctor may recommend keeping such a diary every day for a week, a month, or the duration of your treatment. He or she may review the diary with you to assess your progress, weigh the effectiveness of medications, or make adjustments in your treatment plan. We've included two examples of typical headache diary forms, the simple Headache Diary and the Headache and Medication Log. They vary in terms of how they chart your information, but the goal of both is to uncover a pattern to your migraines and keep a record of their characteristics. Whichever you choose, consider placing it on the bathroom mirror, refrigerator, or some other obvious place as a reminder to fill it out consistently.

Headache and Medication Log

This version of a headache journal looks intimidating at first but is actually quite simple to use and provides a good snapshot of your headaches over a period of time. Before you begin using it, read the explanation of how to fill it out.

HEADACHE AND MEDICATION LOG

NAME: ______________________ MONTH: ______________________ YEAR: ______________

	DATE:	1	2	3	4	5	6	7	8	9	10	11	12	13	14	15	16	17	18	19	20	21	22	23	24	25	26	27	28	29	30	31
HEADACHE INTENSITY	Life-threatening pain	10	10	10	10	10	10	10	10	10	10	10	10	10	10	10	10	10	10	10	10	10	10	10	10	10	10	10	10	10	10	10
	Excruciating pain (ER visit)	9	9	9	9	9	9	9	9	9	9	9	9	9	9	9	9	9	9	9	9	9	9	9	9	9	9	9	9	9	9	9
	Brutal pain (100% bedrest)	8	8	8	8	8	8	8	8	8	8	8	8	8	8	8	8	8	8	8	8	8	8	8	8	8	8	8	8	8	8	8
	Severe pain (partial bedrest)	7	7	7	7	7	7	7	7	7	7	7	7	7	7	7	7	7	7	7	7	7	7	7	7	7	7	7	7	7	7	7
	Moderately severe pain	6	6	6	6	6	6	6	6	6	6	6	6	6	6	6	6	6	6	6	6	6	6	6	6	6	6	6	6	6	6	6
	Moderate pain	5	5	5	5	5	5	5	5	5	5	5	5	5	5	5	5	5	5	5	5	5	5	5	5	5	5	5	5	5	5	5
	Light moderate pain	4	4	4	4	4	4	4	4	4	4	4	4	4	4	4	4	4	4	4	4	4	4	4	4	4	4	4	4	4	4	4
	Mild pain	3	3	3	3	3	3	3	3	3	3	3	3	3	3	3	3	3	3	3	3	3	3	3	3	3	3	3	3	3	3	3
	Very mild pain	2	2	2	2	2	2	2	2	2	2	2	2	2	2	2	2	2	2	2	2	2	2	2	2	2	2	2	2	2	2	2
	Light pressure or aura only	1	1	1	1	1	1	1	1	1	1	1	1	1	1	1	1	1	1	1	1	1	1	1	1	1	1	1	1	1	1	1
	No pain at all	0	0	0	0	0	0	0	0	0	0	0	0	0	0	0	0	0	0	0	0	0	0	0	0	0	0	0	0	0	0	0
LENGTH OF HEADACHE (hours)																																
DISABLITY LEVEL	Trip to ER/MD office for RX	4	4	4	4	4	4	4	4	4	4	4	4	4	4	4	4	4	4	4	4	4	4	4	4	4	4	4	4	4	4	4
	Bedrest required	3	3	3	3	3	3	3	3	3	3	3	3	3	3	3	3	3	3	3	3	3	3	3	3	3	3	3	3	3	3	3
	Severely impaired functioning	2	2	2	2	2	2	2	2	2	2	2	2	2	2	2	2	2	2	2	2	2	2	2	2	2	2	2	2	2	2	2
	Mildly impaired functioning	1	1	1	1	1	1	1	1	1	1	1	1	1	1	1	1	1	1	1	1	1	1	1	1	1	1	1	1	1	1	1
	Normal work and function	0	0	0	0	0	0	0	0	0	0	0	0	0	0	0	0	0	0	0	0	0	0	0	0	0	0	0	0	0	0	0

ASSOCIATED SYMPTOMS																															
Sensitive to light	lgts	lgts	lgts	lgts	lgts	lgts	lgts	lgts	lgts	lgts	lgts	lgts	lgts	lgts	lgts	lgts	lgts	lgts	lgts	lgts	lgts	lgts	lgts	lgts	lgts	lgts	lgts	lgts	lgts	lgts	lgts
Sensitive to sound	snd	snd	snd	snd	snd	snd	snd	snd	snd	snd	snd	snd	snd	snd	snd	snd	snd	snd	snd	snd	snd	snd	snd	snd	snd	snd	snd	snd	snd	snd	snd
Nausea	nau	nau	nau	nau	nau	nau	nau	nau	nau	nau	nau	nau	nau	nau	nau	nau	nau	nau	nau	nau	nau	nau	nau	nau	nau	nau	nau	nau	nau	nau	nau
Vomiting	vom	vom	vom	vom	vom	vom	vom	vom	vom	vom	vom	vom	vom	vom	vom	vom	vom	vom	vom	vom	vom	vom	vom	vom	vom	vom	vom	vom	vom	vom	vom
Headache on 1/2 head	1/2	1/2	1/2	1/2	1/2	1/2	1/2	1/2	1/2	1/2	1/2	1/2	1/2	1/2	1/2	1/2	1/2	1/2	1/2	1/2	1/2	1/2	1/2	1/2	1/2	1/2	1/2	1/2	1/2	1/2	1/2
Headache on both sides	both	both	both	both	both	both	both	both	both	both	both	both	both	both	both	both	both	both	both	both	both	both	both	both	both	both	both	both	both	both	both
Throbbing headache	thbg	thbg	thbg	thbg	thbg	thbg	thbg	thbg	thbg	thbg	thbg	thbg	thbg	thbg	thbg	thbg	thbg	thbg	thbg	thbg	thbg	thbg	thbg	thbg	thbg	thbg	thbg	thbg	thbg	thbg	thbg
Steady (light) headache	stdy	stdy	stdy	stdy	stdy	stdy	stdy	stdy	stdy	stdy	stdy	stdy	stdy	stdy	stdy	stdy	stdy	stdy	stdy	stdy	stdy	stdy	stdy	stdy	stdy	stdy	stdy	stdy	stdy	stdy	stdy
Worse with movement	mvt	mvt	mvt	mvt	mvt	mvt	mvt	mvt	mvt	mvt	mvt	mvt	mvt	mvt	mvt	mvt	mvt	mvt	mvt	mvt	mvt	mvt	mvt	mvt	mvt	mvt	mvt	mvt	mvt	mvt	mvt
Migraine aura (visual)	vis	vis	vis	vis	vis	vis	vis	vis	vis	vis	vis	vis	vis	vis	vis	vis	vis	vis	vis	vis	vis	vis	vis	vis	vis	vis	vis	vis	vis	vis	vis
Migraine aura (neurological)	neur	neur	neur	neur	neur	neur	neur	neur	neur	neur	neur	neur	neur	neur	neur	neur	neur	neur	neur	neur	neur	neur	neur	neur	neur	neur	neur	neur	neur	neur	neur
Menstrual period	men	men	men	men	men	men	men	men	men	men	men	men	men	men	men	men	men	men	men	men	men	men	men	men	men	men	men	men	men	men	men
Other (write in comments)	othr	othr	othr	othr	othr	othr	othr	othr	othr	othr	othr	othr	othr	othr	othr	othr	othr	othr	othr	othr	othr	othr	othr	othr	othr	othr	othr	othr	othr	othr	othr

RESCUE MEDICATIONS TAKEN FOR HEADACHE PAIN

Initially, you may find it useful to fill in all of the information to help identify triggers and patterns, but once you have enough information or your headaches are stable, you can simply circle the pain rating each day. Otherwise, you may begin to view it as too much work; at a certain point too much information becomes counterproductive.

1. Fill out each column of the form for every day of the month, even on days when you don't have a headache.
2. HEADACHE INTENSITY: Circle the score number that best describes the PEAK LEVEL ("High Tide") of headache pain reached during the headache on this date. Colored pencil or pen shows up best. A level 9 or 10 headache is a headache that is the worst pain imaginable. Days that are totally headache free should be scored level 0. Using your best judgment and personal pain tolerance, choose any number between 0 and 10 that you feel best represents the intensity of your headache.
3. LENGTH OF HEADACHE: Record the total duration of the headache (in hours) in this box. If the headache lasts for several days and nights, record "24" in several boxes in a row, one for each day of pain.

4. DISABILITY LEVEL: Circle the level corresponding to the MAXIMUM level of disability caused by the headache. Level 3, for example, means that you had to go to bed for some time during the day.
5. ASSOCIATED SYMPTOMS: Circle the code letters corresponding to symptoms that precede or accompany the headache. For example, "neur" means that neurological symptoms such as weakness or numbness of part of your body was associated with the headache. Circle "men" on each day you have a menstrual period.
6. MEDICATIONS TAKEN: List on the lines any abortive medications taken during the headache. Do not list daily preventive medication taken for headache, and do not list medication taken for any reason other than a headache. Opposite these medications, record in the boxes for each headache how many tablets were taken during the entire day. For example, if four Advil are taken for a headache on April 4, write "Advil" on the first line at left, then move across columns until the headache for April 4 and record "4" in that box.

Simple Headache Diary			
This diary form is fairly self-explanatory. Simply fill in the chart each time you have a headache. If you have more than three episodes in a time period, you will need to reproduce this sheet multiple times.			
	First episode	Second episode	Third episode
Date/day of the week of headache			
Time of onset			
Time of resolution			
Warning signs			
Location(s) of the pain			
Type of pain (e.g. sharp, dull, steady, throb)			
Maximum intensity of the pain*			
Additional symptoms			
Activities/circumstances at time of onset			
Time of most recent meal prior to onset			

	First episode	Second episode	Third episode
Food/drink most recently consumed prior to onset			
Medication(s) taken for headache			
Response to medication(s)			
Other action(s) taken for relief			
Response to action(s)			
Last menstrual period**			
Medication(s) currently taken for other condition(s)			
*on a scale from 1 to 10, with 1 being very mild pain and 10 being the worst pain possible **beginning date and ending date			
Note: Permission is granted to reproduce this page of the report for individual use.			

Headache History

A diary can be useful for helping your doctor determine your current pattern of headaches. Also, many patients feel a sense of empowerment when they track their headaches because it makes them feel like they are taking control of the situation. We applaud the effort and certainly welcome when our patients bring such a tool to an appointment. In deciding whether someone needs daily preventive treatment to decrease the number of headaches, the headache diary provides reliable information about the average number of headache days per month. (Typically, we will offer preventive treatment if patients are routinely having one or more headaches a week. When headaches are less frequent, treatment of individual episodes alone may be sufficient.) However, a timeline of headaches does not give us the entire story.

Your doctor will find having a summary of your entire headache history to be one of the most useful tools for getting to the heart of the matter. A complete overview of your situation tells your doctor what has already been done and provides clues for possible next steps. For example, in trying to address Leslie's concerns about whether her headaches are the symptom of some underlying medical condition, we will need to take a complete medical history and perform a physical exam. If need be, we may order some tests. During this process, we ask a series of questions like the ones included below. Take some time to consider these questions before your doctor's visit; this will enable you to think through the answers and give as accurate a representation of your problem as possible.

- What made you seek medical attention?
- When did your headaches begin?
- Does anything seem related to their onset?
- How often do they occur?
- How long do they last?
- When do they occur?
- Where is the pain located?
- How severe is it?
- What does it feel like?
- Do you notice any other symptoms before or during the headaches?
- Does anything seem to trigger or worsen the headaches?
- Does anything ease the pain?
- Does anyone in your family have a history of headaches?
- How is your family and work life?
- How have your headaches affected your life?
- What treatments have been tried for your headaches, and how effective have they been? This includes nondrug treatments such as acupuncture, herbs, or vitamins. The more details you provide here, including doses and length of treatment, the better.
- What other medical problems do you have, and how are they being treated? This can affect the

treatments a doctor may choose for your headache problem or provide important clues to possible medical causes of the headaches.

Next Steps

Once you're armed with good information about your migraines, you need to consider what to do with it. Who have you prepared these questions for? Which doctor is best equipped to deal with your issues? Many people start with their primary-care or family doctor. This can be a good first step, but not all doctors are equally versed in headache treatment, and some may not be equipped to give you as much help as you need. Be persistent. If after a reasonable period of time and several treatment attempts, you aren't getting better, or your doctor doesn't seem to be taking your problem seriously, consider seeing a neurologist or headache specialist.

chapter 5

Finding the Right Doctor

Seeing a doctor for your headaches the first time is a bit like going out on a blind date: There's no guarantee that even a highly recommended doctor will be right for you. One reason for this—perhaps the biggest reason—is that people have different expectations about what they're looking for in a doctor.

Charlotte, for instance, went to a headache specialist she felt had helped her a great deal; he was patient, a good listener, and seemed sympathetic to her ongoing struggle with migraines. When her friend Pam, who also suffered from migraines, asked her for a recommendation, she didn't hesitate to give her the specialist's number. Unfortunately, the doctor didn't turn out to be a good fit for Pam. His location was inconvenient, and she was annoyed that she had to wait two weeks for an appointment. She also felt he wasn't aggressive enough in his treatment approach.

In our view, the definition of *good doctor* starts with knowing what you value most. If you could have it all, what qualities would your doctor possess? For people like Charlotte, it's all about bedside manner, personality, and communication skills. Other people value smarts, technical skills, or expertise. Still others rely on credentials, such as where a doctor went to medical school or received residency training. Patients like Pam care most about how the office runs, how quickly the phone is answered, or how friendly the receptionist is. A little forethought and some research can help you crystallize your priorities and narrow your choices down for the best options.

Starting with Primary Care

A good place to start your doctor search is with your primary-care physician. This is especially true in areas where certified headache specialists are few and far between. Although most primary-care practitioners aren't headache specialists per se, some may have quite a bit of experience with headache management or at least have an interest in treating patients who suffer from migraines.

Your primary-care practitioner may suggest a preliminary course of action before sending you to a specialist or may immediately refer you on. A good primary-care practitioner will concede when they aren't able to do justice to your condition and help you find the right expert, typically a neurologist or board-certified headache specialist. Some people don't put much faith in their primary care's opinion and want a referral right away. We think that's unfortunate because many primary-care doctors and nurse-practitioners do an excellent job with headache problems. Consider working with your primary-care provider to address your problem if she shows the interest and seems knowledgeable. If she seems dismissive of your symptoms or treatment recommendations aren't helping, it's probably best to move on.

Even if you do decide to seek help elsewhere, we recommend keeping your primary-care doctor in the loop. For patients with severe headaches, a primary-care physician can play a significant role in coordinating overall medical care; as your "gate keeper," he or she has the best understanding of your overall health and is in the best position to balance your headache care with the rest of your health care. Also, as treatment progresses, many patients wind

The Exclusive Language of Your Doctor

During your doctor's visit, you may spend a lot of time talking about the things that aren't causing your headaches—and you may even leave the office before realizing you never really got the answer about what *is* causing them. After reviewing the details of your symptoms and performing an examination, your doctor may describe some possible causes and whittle them down to only one or two things, not because there are definite findings or test results indicating the diagnosis but because the other explanations don't seem likely for one reason or another.

An underappreciated but undeniable truth in medical practice is that frequently we can more reliably tell what the problem is not than what it is. By the end of your visit, your doctor may suspect that you do indeed have migraines. However, this and many other headache diagnoses are based on clinical information: There are no accurate or specific tests that "prove" someone has migraines. Ruling out other possibilities (by using your description of symptoms and other medical history, physical examination, and sometimes testing), is important—in fact, critical—in determining this diagnosis. Sometimes the cause of your headaches can never be proven. A diagnosis of possible migraine headaches along with reassurance that dangerous causes of headaches have been excluded may seem less definitive than a diagnosis that can be proven. Often, though, patients find that reassurance about conditions they don't have may wind up being the most helpful and reassuring thing their doctor can do for them.

up getting prescription refills from their primary-care physician rather than the specialist.

Other Referral Sources

If your primary-care provider doesn't have a suitable treatment or referral for you, another good place to find recommendations is your insurance provider. They'll often have lists of headache specialists on their Web sites or available on their hotlines. Most states have a list of licensed physicians online, with information about medical training and board certification; these can be valuable because they also offer information about malpractice claims and disciplinary actions against doctors, which you may want to check before you make an appointment.

There are also several excellent online resources we

recommend: The American Council for Headache Education's Web site has a searchable online database of doctors who belong to the organization. The United Council for Neurologic Subspecialties Web site lists physicians who are certified in Headache Medicine; at the time of this writing, there are just a few hundred of these specialists nationwide, but numbers are growing. The certification is relatively new, so you shouldn't necessarily consider it as a negative if your doctor doesn't have this credential.

The National Headache Foundation Web site provides contact information for doctors who have special qualifications in headache management. To be included, doctors have to devote a substantial portion of their practice to headache patients or research, have published an article in a peer-reviewed journal, completed fifty continuing-medical-education credit hours in headache in the last five years, presented at scientific meetings or published articles on headache, and been involved in teaching lecturing, publication, or research in the last seven years. (For a complete list of resources see chapter 14.)

Do keep in mind that just because a doctor is on a list doesn't mean that you'll like him or her or be satisfied with the treatment you receive. And you may find a doctor who isn't on any list but who you believe will be the best person to treat your headaches. As we mentioned previously, doctors identified as headache specialists are sparse in some areas; patients in some areas of the country should be prepared to travel if they need to see one.

It also makes sense to ask fellow headache suffers for referrals. As Pam discovered, it doesn't always work out, but it's at least worth asking around. If the same doctor's name is mentioned over and over again, it's a good sign that you're on the right track. You can also look for referrals on Web site message boards run by support groups or organizations with a special interest in migraines. Proceed with caution on the recommendations and advice you find on them, though. Online message boards often don't have regular administrators, and the conversations aren't always policed by a knowledgeable medical professional. You should thoroughly vet the information you find through those sources.

Finally, it's worth noting that we've known patients with chronic headaches who have searched the medical literature to find an expert who is doing research or setting standards of treatment on their particular condition. Often these individuals have already seen several doctors and haven't found relief. Some of these patients will even get on a plane and travel across the country for an appointment with someone they consider a guru. We agree that keeping up with the latest science on migraines is a

Why Your Doctor Sometimes Tells You "No"

Perhaps you read a newspaper article describing a headache treatment studied by a highly reputable academic medical center. It sounded so good, so safe, so appropriate for you that you can't imagine why your doctor would say "no" or suggest something else.

Although it is not always easy, doctors must learn to say no, and they are taught to do so in medical school and during later training. Given all the direct-to-consumer marketing, it's easy to believe that everything you see in the media works miracles. But clearly, every person with a headache does not require an MRI, neurological consultation, or the latest medication. Despite what you read or see on TV, do keep in mind that there may be good reasons for what your doctor is saying even when you aren't getting what you expected. If you don't understand why the doctor is reluctant to prescribe the medication you expected or recommend the test you thought you needed, ask for an explanation. Understanding the reasoning can be helpful not only as a way to be better informed about your condition but also to avoid misunderstanding.

Ideally, decisions about how best to treat your migraines will be shared between you and your doctor. Studies show that many people are ready to switch doctors if they don't get what they want or expect, and that would be a shame if you have a good relationship with your doctor otherwise. Don't be afraid to ask your doctor to explain recommendations, especially when they do not match your expectations; it may be the only way to really understand what your doctor is saying.

wise idea. And, of course, everyone wants the best medical care possible. But in our experience, a long-distance relationship with a doctor is not ideal for ongoing care. While it may be valuable to seek a consultation from the best experts in the field no matter where they're located, you're almost always better off finding a local treatment provider to see on a regular basis.

chapter 6

Your Doctor's Appointment

Adrianna had been living on over-the-counter medications to cope with her migraines for several years. Once they stopped working for her, and the frequency and intensity of her headaches began escalating, she finally decided it was time to see a doctor. She started with her primary-care physician, who, when treatment was not successful, referred her to one neurologist, then another. None of their recommended treatments helped get her migraines under control. Now that she's about to see her fourth doctor, she's feeling a bit discouraged. She's tired of wasting time and energy; she wants relief, and she wants it now.

This is a common scenario for migraine sufferers. It's

not that doctors don't care about your suffering. Some are simply not equipped to deal with patients with migraines. Even if they are, they aren't always the best fit in other ways. Added to that is the fact that even the best available treatment for migraine does not work for everyone.

What should your expectations be? How can you tell if a doctor is right for you? What questions should you be asking your doctor—and what questions should your doctor be asking you? With some forethought and preparation, you can prepare for your first visit with a doctor to ensure it's as productive as possible and to help determine whether or not you've found a good match.

Your First Visit

Think of your first visit as an interview. Begin by learning what the doctor's treatment philosophies are and what kind of relationships he has with his patients. You don't need to be defensive or conduct an interrogation but it's essential to gather information about what's important to you. If a doctor isn't going to work out, it's better to know sooner than later.

You can ask questions at the beginning of your appointment, as you go along, or at the end of your appointment.

Just make sure you feel satisfied with both the answers and how the responses are given. A doctor who is skilled and knowledgeable and yet comes off as annoyed, offended, or condescending—or who simply won't take the time to answer your questions—is not likely to be a good fit in the long run. (Refer to the "Questions to Ask Your Doctor" on page 81 to help formulate your list of questions.)

Part of the treatment experience is how you'll be treated by the office staff, so be sure to consider this as part of your appraisal. Note whether the staff is pleasant and treats you with respect and how long the doctor keeps you waiting. Even if you love your doctor, you may not tolerate two hours in the waiting room. You'll also want to clarify how the doctor handles things like follow-up visits, phone calls, and prescription requests and familiarize yourself with phone-call-return policies, how often you'll be seen, and whether or not your doctor makes trips to the emergency room.

Of course, a good doctor will also ask *you* questions to learn the specifics of your migraines and medical history. Typically, a specialist will explore other symptoms linked to your headaches and whether other family members have problem headaches plus review information about the location, frequency, and other characteristics of your headaches, as well as your sleep habits, family history, and other potential headache triggers. An accurate, detailed description of your symptoms is invaluable, so come ready to discuss when your headaches began, what they feel like, and particular situations that seem to prompt or worsen them. Most headache specialists review previous and present headache therapies for a closer look at what's worked for you and what hasn't. All of these questions can reveal potential treatment options and help determine whether further testing is merited.

Most surprising to many patients is that they've come to talk about how painful their migraines are, but their doctor seems more interested in how much the headaches interfere with their lives. Of course, a good doctor should be sympathetic to your suffering, but they're aware that every individual perceives pain differently; some people can power through even when they are in the throes of a real pounder while others take to their bed at the first throb they feel in their temple. Since there is no accurate way to categorize pain severity, a more reliable measure for your doctor to evaluate is disability.

Understanding how often headaches sideline you and prevent you from functioning normally provides valuable clues on how to treat you. If you've filled out a headache diary, and your doctor doesn't seem all that interested, this is not necessarily something to hold against him.

Although in our practice we believe it is important to take the time to review a diary if someone has taken the trouble to keep one, we don't consider the information as important as the information we get from having an in-depth conversation. Many doctors also rely on tools, questionnaires, and surveys that help measure the impact your headaches have on your life over a specific period of time rather than a journal.

Also, don't be put off if your doctor does a psychological assessment or asks about a history of sexual, physical, or verbal abuse. Migraines are often associated or accompanied by certain psychological conditions such as depression or stress, and abuse victims frequently experience migraines; a doctor who asks about these things deserves points for being thorough.

The Physical Exam

A physical exam is a must at your first visit and should include a blood-pressure check and a careful look inside your eyes with an ophthalmoscope. Increased pressure in the head, which can be a sign of a brain tumor, can cause swelling of the optic nerve; the ophthalmoscope examination can reveal such swelling. In some people, tension and migraine headaches produce telltale signs such as spasms in the neck and shoulder muscles or even tender areas in the muscle that can sometimes be felt as a nodule or tight band of tissue—your doctor should check for these. In most people who have tension or migraine headaches, the physical examination doesn't turn up anything unusual—which means that your headaches aren't the result of some underlying medical condition. That should be a relief.

We encourage everyone over the age of forty to have regular appointments with an eye doctor to be checked for glaucoma. This condition, which involves elevated pressure in the eye, can cause headachelike pain. Glaucoma is treatable, but it can lead to blindness if it goes undetected. Because eyestrain from squinting can occasionally cause headaches, a thorough eye exam may also reveal that something as simple as getting new glasses might alleviate your pain.

Questions to Ask Your Doctor

- How long have you been treating headache patients?
- Any special interest or training in headache? What if I need help after office hours? Patients should get information about the policy on office visits, phone calls, Rx refills, etc. from the get-go. These things loom large in the life of a headache patient. (Often these details will be covered in the introductory information mailed to the patient or available on the office's Web site.)
- What tests will you do to diagnose the cause of my headaches? How accurate are the tests? How safe are the tests?
- Will you or your staff answer my questions about the diagnosis?
- Do you have a plan of treatment if the first two or three recommendations fail?
- Will you follow through with your recommendations until we reach an optimal level of therapy?
- What treatments other than medication do you think may help me (e.g. acupuncture, massage, physical therapy, diet modification, exercise, etc.)?
- Are you willing to work as a team with me and other health-care providers, such as practitioners of complementary and alternative therapies, a chronic-illness counselor, a mental-health provider, and a pain specialist?

Questions Your Doctor Will Ask You

Before an appointment, jot down the answers to these questions:

- When did your headaches begin?
- Does anything seem related to their onset?
- How often do they occur?
- How long do they last?
- When do they occur?
- Where is the pain located?
- How severe and debilitating is the pain?
- Do you notice any other symptoms before or during the headaches?
- Does anything seem to trigger or worsen the headaches?
- Does anything ease the pain?
- Does anyone in your family have a history of headaches?
- How is your family and work life?
- How have your headaches affected your life?
- What have you used in the past to treat your headaches? (Be as detailed as possible about the names and doses of the treatments and how long you took them.)

Diagnostic Testing

Considering how common headaches are and the long list of potential causes, remarkably few people require any diagnostic tests. In fact, there are no special tests that specifically diagnose migraines. A doctor usually arrives at a diagnosis of migraine based on your history and symptoms. As we mentioned, in most cases a physical and neurological examination will be entirely normal. Additional testing usually isn't warranted unless your headaches have features that are not typical for migraines, you develop other worrisome symptoms, or if there is any doubt about your diagnosis.

People with a long history of headaches that haven't changed much in intensity or frequency are less likely to need additional tests than individuals just starting to experience headaches or whose headaches have gotten worse, or otherwise have changed dramatically. If there is some unexplained abnormality noted on your neurological examination, testing may be warranted. If your doctor decides on further testing, it will usually be a CT scan—short for computed tomography and often pronounced "cat scan"—or a magnetic resonance imaging (MRI) scan. A CT scan is taken by a special X-ray machine. In some cases, a contrast dye is administered intravenously to define the brain structures more clearly. Rather than sending one wide

X-ray beam through your body, this machine sends out many beams from many angles. A computer uses the results to generate detailed, cross-sectional pictures of your body. This test provides a much clearer picture of your head than a regular X-ray.

For an MRI scan, you'll be placed inside a machine that can be likened to a large, well-lit tube. The process is noisy, so you must wear ear protection. Some people feel claustrophobic inside the device, but many testing facilities provide earphones so you can listen to music to ease some of the anxiety. MRI machines of a more open design are available in some facilities. The procedure takes twenty to forty-five minutes. If intravenous dye is needed to enhance the image, it's usually given halfway through the procedure. You may feel nervous or uncomfortable at the mere thought of such a test, but keep in mind that it's a painless yet valuable way for identifying tumors, bleeding, areas of damaged brain tissue, and even sinus infections.

Although magnetic resonance imaging (MRI) creates an image similar to that produced by a CT scan, the technique is quite different. Rather than using X-rays, the MRI machine relies on a strong magnetic field. Tissues give off minute electromagnetic waves in frequencies that differ according to the type involved. A computer tallies the vibrations and uses this data to create cross-sectional images on many different planes. These remarkably detailed pictures can show the difference between brain tissue and tumors and highlight areas of the brain that have been damaged by a stroke or other neurological conditions.

There is significant overlap in the information obtained by each of these studies; however, there are also important differences. In many situations, there is no clear superiority of one over the other, but as a general rule most headache experts think that MRI does a better job of evaluating a number of possible causes of headache and prefer it. An additional worry is that CT scans involve radiation, and doctors are becoming more cautious about exposing patients to unneeded radiation.

Summing Up Your Visit

Success with headache treatment may not come overnight. Clinically comprehensive treatment, from initial consultations through comprehensive evaluations and complete implementation, could take a number of months and visits. This highly individualized approach has only one goal in mind: to determine the cause of your headache pain and give you a plan to help prevent and manage it.

And, while you should expect results from treatment, don't expect miracles. Patients who've had frequent headaches over a long period of time can become passive and begin to view their doctor as a savior. This isn't realistic. The idea is to develop a plan, try the plan, then come back to review how the plan is working. Unreasonable expectations lead to dissatisfaction with almost any doctor, even one who is trying hard to solve your problems. That said, your doctor should listen to your concerns rather than brush you off dismissively. At minimum, your doctor should be knowledgeable about proper diagnosis and treatment of migraines and willing to try new things if the first course of action doesn't work.

After your initial visit, you may have some concerns. If you're generally happy with the doctor and practice, you might try discussing your concerns. If you get a proactive response, then it's more likely your needs will be met. If not, you always have the option of moving on.

Since headaches are a condition of long duration, treatment is usually a work in progress. Both you and your doctor must be willing to go through the process. Because of the complexity of headaches, your doctor may recommend more than one treatment or change your treatment depending on the results. Each person's headache has its own characteristics and may be managed in a different way. We'll discuss mapping out a treatment plan in upcoming chapters.

chapter 7

Special Cases

Although migraines are typically thought of as a "woman's disease," this is not always the case. People of both sexes, of all ages, and all walks of life can suffer from chronic headaches. Migraines sometimes catch women off guard, too, striking them unexpectedly during pregnancy or as they enter menopause. This chapter provides a brief overview of how different groups can be affected by migraine headaches.

Women and Migraines

During childhood, boys are slightly more likely than girls to have headaches. But after puberty, the situation reverses, with women much more likely to experience migraine headaches. These numbers are even higher for women during their childbearing years, where up to a third of women followed for a year will experience the severe headache typical of a migraine. What makes women so susceptible to chronic, pounding headaches during the reproductive time of their life? The answer differs depending upon what stage of life they are in but it can often be traced to one aspect of their biology: cycling female hormones.

Menstrual Migraines

Hormonal fluctuations that occur as part of a woman's monthly menstrual cycle can aggravate any inherited tendency to migraines, probably by making it easier for headaches to occur in the first place and perhaps by making those headaches more severe or longer lasting.

Fluctuations in estrogen levels have long been linked to headaches. Women are more likely to experience migraines and other kinds of headaches during menstruation and the days leading up to it. Research is conflicting about whether a migraine is more likely around the time of ovulation (see Figure 5). For some women, migraine headaches that occur in the days before menstruation tend to be particularly severe and incapacitating. They can be more persistent, too, sometimes lasting for days.

Some researchers believe that estrogen affects pain pathways by influencing levels of brain chemicals (neurotransmitters) or the response that the brain has to them. Estrogen receptors are found in the brain, and estrogen is known to cause inflammation and influence pain perception. Others suspect that estrogen withdrawal triggers migraine headaches, perhaps by altering the balance in the brain between factors that promote a headache and those that work against it.

Menstrual migraine headaches can be treated like any other migraine headaches. For many women, aspirin or another NSAID, such as ibuprofen, or typical migraine treatments such as the triptan medications, work well and can be used on an as-needed basis. If this approach fails, NSAIDs such as aspirin or naproxen may be taken daily, beginning a few days before the attack is suspected and continuing for a total of five to seven days.

There is some evidence that taking triptans daily in this way (for example, frovatriptan 2.5 mg twice a day) can be helpful, but this method of treatment is not approved by the U.S. Food and Drug Administration (FDA). Nevertheless, it is something we are willing to try for women who don't get relief from more conventional treatments.

Since this kind of scheduled treatment is only effective for women whose periods and headache cycles are highly predictable, we usually reserve it for women who experience their menstrual-related migraine attacks in a predictable relationship to the menstrual flow.

Women with migraines often wonder if they can use birth-control pills or patches that contain estrogen. In some cases, they have been told that "the pill" shouldn't be used by anyone with migraines because it can cause strokes. Or they may have heard that it will make their headaches worse. The first of these matters has to do with safety, and the second has to do with how well the treatment is tolerated; in other words, side effects.

Let's take the safety question first. Nearly all forms of birth control carry risks. Birth control methods such as the pill or patch that contain hormones—especially those that contain a combination of estrogen and progesterone, often referred to as *combination contraceptives*—are the most effective method of birth control.

Birth-control methods that contain estrogen are known to increase the risk of blood clots and stroke. This increased risk is very small for most women and often worth taking in exchange for reliable protection from pregnancy. However, women who have migraine with aura seem to be one group (along with women who smoke or have high blood pressure) where the stroke risk is higher, and many experts worry that the combined risk (from aura and from estrogen) is too high. For this reason, we advise caution when taking any sort of estrogen-containing birth-control method for women who have aura. (See chapter 2 for the definition of aura.) Most experts don't feel that women who have migraines without aura and are under thirty-five need to avoid the pill or patch. Progesterone-only methods of birth control are also available, but are not quite as effective and can have other side effects—but they are a safe alternative for women with migraines who can't or don't want to use estrogen. The matter of birth-control safety and migraines is definitely something to discuss with your doctor.

Safety is one thing. Side effects are another. The side effect we worry about with estrogen-containing contraception is worsening of headaches. In our experience, it's difficult to predict whether an individual woman with migraines will experience an increase in headache frequency or intensity when she begins taking the combination contraceptive pill or patch. When this does happen, it usually occurs during the placebo week, when the pills don't contain any estrogen or when the patch is removed. There is some evidence that continuous use of the patch form of estrogen-containing birth control (with no break from hormones as in the usual pill regimen) may decrease the intensity of menstrual migraine headaches compared to headaches in women who take the pill in the usual way. We've also had success using the contraceptive pill in this way. However, in the study that looked at this matter, the difference in headache intensity between the two groups was very small.

In our experience, women with migraines vary in their response to birth-control methods that contain hormones. Some clearly worsen while others notice no big changes in headaches. Because scientific evidence about the effects of birth control on headaches is conflicting, trial and error may be necessary to see what holds true for you. Many practitioners find that, despite what the research says, some of their female patients actually report improvement when they begin taking estrogen-containing contraceptives. This underscores the need to stay open-minded when trying to find what works best in each particular case.

In most cases, the benefits of effective hormonal birth control (reliable prevention of pregnancy, decreases in anemia, and control of endometriosis) must be weighed against potential problems (worsening of headache, risk of blood clots and stroke). There is no one right answer for everyone.

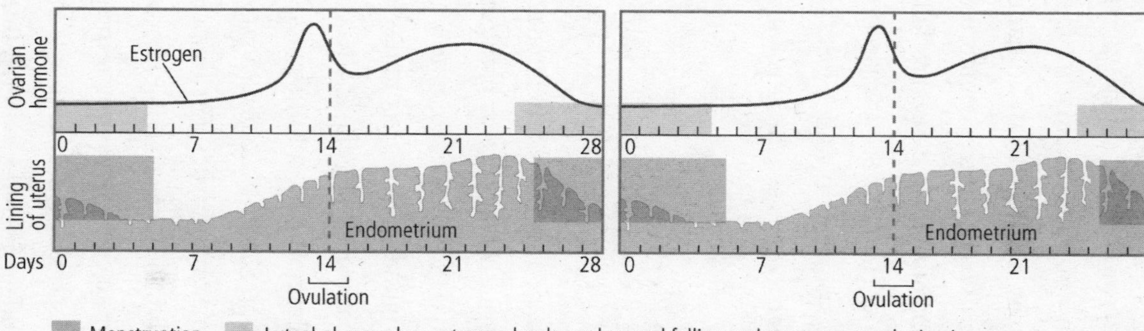

Figure 5: Menstrual migraine

Around the time of menopause, many women experience a gradual improvement in previously troublesome headaches. Women who had particular trouble with menstrual migraines may be most likely to experience this improvement. The use of estrogen-containing hormone-replacement therapy after menopause has fallen from favor because of worries about heart disease, breast cancer, and stroke. Many women also find it may increase the frequency and intensity of headache attacks.

Migraines During Pregnancy

We tell our patients of childbearing years to be careful about getting pregnant if they are on migraine medications that carry risks for either mother or child or where the risks are unknown. For migraine patients actively trying to conceive, we recommend they discontinue taking medication if at all possible. There's no evidence that there needs to be a cooling-off period from migraine medications before getting pregnant, so women can try to conceive as soon as they come off the drugs. For women who aren't able to step off medication completely, we choose drugs that are least likely to cause problems during pregnancy and give them the lowest doses possible.

For patients undergoing infertility treatments, it's important to know that headaches are a common side effect, especially for women who—surprise, surprise—already have migraines to begin with. Several reports suggest that Clomiphene®, a drug used in some infertility regimens, ups the incidence of migraines.

We advise all women of childbearing age to take a daily folic-acid supplement of at least 400 micrograms (0.4 milligrams) to reduce the risk of birth defects. Folic-acid supplementation is especially important for women using headache medications that contain barbiturates and divalproex sodium, which may interfere with folate metabolism.

High, stable levels of estrogen associated with pregnancy appear to have a beneficial effect on migraines. The majority of women who have migraines report feeling better during pregnancy. However, there are exceptions to this rule.

Women who have migraines without aura are more likely to improve with pregnancy than are those who have aura, and women whose headaches seemed to be linked with their menstrual cycle are also more likely to get some relief. Aura may also appear for the first time during pregnancy. If headaches don't improve by the end of the first trimester, it's unlikely they will. If that is the case, we see no reason to withhold treatment from someone with severe headaches.

In general, pregnant women have fewer treatment options. Migraines can sometimes be difficult to distinguish from dangerous causes of headaches that are more common in pregnancy and postpartum. Migraines are also a risk factor for several serious pregnancy complications.

In general, women with migraines don't appear to have a significantly increased risk of giving birth to infants with congenital defects or other problems. However, reasonably good evidence does suggest they may be at risk for more complications during pregnancy. For example, migraines can elevate the risk of preeclampsia, dangerously high blood pressure that occurs during pregnancy, which is in turn associated with an increased risk of placental abruption, seizures, and stroke. The risk of preeclampsia in migraineurs appears to increase in proportion to the severity of the headaches and may appear earlier and be more critical in women who have migraines than in those who do not.

Many pregnant or lactating migraineurs take their medication whenever they have individual headache attacks while some also need preventive treatment as well. In general, we recommend limiting medication as much as possible and defaulting to other approaches when feasible (see chapter 9 for alternative treatments and chapter 10 for lifestyle changes). Appropriate treatment choices also vary with the stage of pregnancy, and may differ for pregnancy and lactation. Your doctor should make a thorough evaluation of your personal situation to guide decisions about how to treat your migraines.

Postpartum headaches are extremely common, with more than a third of women experiencing them during the six weeks after delivery, and in about half of women who have a prior history of headaches. In one large study, 75 percent of headaches were classifiable as primary headaches like migraines, and just 4 percent were reported to be "incapacitating."

Menopausal Migraines

Women who experience menstrual migraines often pray for menopause! It's their hope that as go their periods, so go their head pains. In many cases, that proves to be true. Over 70 percent of women will see an improvement in their migraines after menopause. The other 30 percent report their migraines are the same or perhaps slightly worse. A very small percentage of women have a new onset of migraines after menopause. Studies show that even after age fifty-five, migraines are still more prevalent in women than in men. This makes some researchers suspect that hormone-related effects on the brain may persist after menopause. The stage of a woman's life dubbed perimenopause refers to the entire period of major hormonal changes during which some but not all women experience hot flashes, emotional turmoil, and night sweats. These will usually lessen over time once the hormonal transition is complete, e.g. menopause, which is characterized by at least twelve months without a period.

During perimenopause, some women who are prone to migraines are in for a rough go. The cause of migraines in these years can largely be blamed on those pesky hormones. The estrogen cycle may become irregular, causing higher peak estrogen levels; this hormonal rise and fall seems to sensitize the nervous system and incite headaches. The result in some cases is a whopper of a headache, usually during a time when estrogen levels are declining after a prolonged period of elevation.

Our first-line treatment of hormonally triggered migraines doesn't involve hormonal manipulation. Rather, we usually recommend to our patients the same abortive and preventive agents used to treat any other migraine. Many doctors still recommend hormonal-replacement therapy (HRT) to deal with symptoms of menopause, but women with migraines should proceed with caution on this front. Some evidence suggests HRT can make headaches much worse, and it may increase the risk of stroke or cardiovascular problems—women suffering from migraine with aura may already be at increased risk of these things.

Men and Migraines

For most men, an occasional headache is nothing more than a speed bump in the course of a busy day. But for Jason, headaches are a bigger problem. The several head-splitting migraines he experiences each week often cause him to miss work and family time. He frequently tries to tough it out and live with the pain. After all, it isn't the "macho" knee pain or back stiffness his friends complain about after a game of basketball—and even his primary-care doctor has discounted his head pain, telling him men rarely have migraines and that all he needs is a little more sleep and a little less stress.

While it's true that the vast majority of migraine sufferers are women, in the course of a year, about 6 percent of men will have at least one migraine. Even when they finally relent and see a doctor, they're misdiagnosed up to 70 percent of the time. It's easy to see why. Jason listed his symptoms as a one-sided headache with nasal congestion and tearing in one eye. He didn't mention what many doctors think of as the classical migraine symptoms of nausea, vomiting, and sensitivity to light and sound.

Because his primary-care physician isn't especially familiar with migraines and hasn't had a chance to step back to review the big picture of what's going on, he's thinking that Jason might have allergies or a sinus infection. An experienced headache specialist would be more likely to delve deeper into his medical history, perhaps asking about things like family history of migraines and childhood car sickness. This is because research shows that although migraines are common in men, men with migraines aren't as likely as women with migraines to report "classic" associated symptoms of migraines such as nausea, vomiting, and sensitivity to light or noise. Add to that the fact that migraines have a reputation for being a woman's problem, it isn't surprising that men with migraines can have a hard time getting the right diagnosis. (By the way, although men on *average* have fewer problems with migraines than women, this average isn't necessarily true for an *individual* man. We have many male patients with very severe migraines and many female patients whose headaches are less severe.)

Men and Cluster Headaches

Once a migraine is diagnosed, a headache specialist will work with male patients like Jason on managing his triggers, and if he has more than a couple of headaches a week, they'll consider prescribing preventive medication. Prescription medications for individual headache attacks may also be needed. Although in general, men and women don't differ in their responses to medications, men are more prone to cardiovascular problems than women, so drugs that can aggravate this problem might need to be avoided. For example, in older men with a history of heart problems, commonly used migraine-treatment drugs like triptans may not be a good choice since they can affect blood flow to the heart as well as the head. This means that anyone with coronary artery disease or major heart disease risk factors should not use them. Some doctors prescribe antinausea medication, stronger prescription painkillers, or even a short course of steroids for men if their migraines are particularly intense and triptans cannot be used, as they do for women in the same situation.

One headache pattern seen more commonly in men, though by no means exclusively, is known as the cluster headache. Cluster headaches are relatively rare compared to migraines, but this is partly because migraines are so common. Cluster headaches are relatively common, for example, compared with another neurologic condition, multiple sclerosis, that seems prevalent because it gets so much press. Cluster headaches are five to nine times more common in men than women. Cluster headaches are just what they sound like: they cluster over a period of time; they may appear suddenly, occur one or more times daily for weeks at a time only to then disappear altogether. In between, a patient is often completely headache-free. However, the same time the following year— often in the spring or fall—the headaches strike again without warning.

By definition, a cluster headache is a severe but shorter-lasting one-sided headache, usually centering around the eye. The pain is always accompanied by one or more of the following: swelling or tearing of the eye or a runny nose, all on the same side as the headache. During a headache, the patient can be agitated and restless; some even strike their heads against a wall in frustration. In contrast, a migraine patient will usually seek a quiet, dark, restful place.

You might think this dramatic and characteristic pattern would be easy to recognize and diagnose. Studies indicate just the opposite. It's often misdiagnosed and confused with sinus disease or dental problems. It can be many years before the issue is clarified. Many patients by that point have undergone unnecessary dental work or other procedures in their quest for relief.

Whether this is a form of migraine or a completely separate condition is an unsettled question. Special imaging studies suggest that the source of cluster headaches may be in the hypothalamus area of the brain, and this is one finding, among many, that would seem to separate cluster headaches from migraines. There is sure to be more to the story as research progresses.

Treatment of such a severe headache can certainly be challenging. Some medications may stop a cluster episode in its tracks. Other medications may prevent the cluster episodes altogether, or at least blunt the attack. Some treatments may seem a bit unorthodox; for example, when oxygen (breathed by mask from a tank in the home) is mentioned in headache management, it is usually in reference to cluster headaches.

Though it's often a taboo subject for men, they must understand that chronic or disabling headaches are a serious health issue that requires medical attention. They don't have to suck it up or suffer in silence. Just like any other headache sufferer, they owe it to themselves to seek out proper treatment and get relief. This means working with a trained and skilled doctor who understands how to treat migraines and doesn't automatically dismiss any man who walks through the door with a headache.

Children and Migraines

Did you know that children can have migraines? Melissa didn't. She couldn't understand why her four-year-old son James sometimes became sensitive to lights and sounds and complained of dizziness. Though ordinarily an active child, he would become sluggish and sleep for hours when the symptoms hit him. When the pediatrician diagnosed her young son with migraines, Melissa was shocked.

Ten percent of children between the ages of five and fifteen have migraines, and 28 percent of adolescents between the ages of fifteen and nineteen experience migraine attacks. More than a fifth of juvenile migraine sufferers experience their first migraine before the age of five. Migraine attacks begin at an earlier age for boys than girls, but girls are more likely to develop migraine attacks after puberty.

In addition to the symptoms James describes, preschool-aged children may cry, rock back and forth, and become irritable when they're in the midst of a migraine. It's a particular challenge for them since they sometimes don't understand or are often unable to express what they're feeling. In our experience, vomiting is often a prominent part of migraines in children, and (mercifully) children's migraines often are shorter than those experienced by adults. Children with headaches frequently show a strong desire to go to sleep, and often this is an effective way of ending a headache rather than the use of medication. Regardless of age, migraines can be heartbreakingly debilitating for youngsters; attacks can interfere with their social life, and they tend to miss a lot of school.

A child's migraines will often have an identifiable hereditary component. Are you or someone in your immediate family also susceptible to migraines? Potential triggers include bright lights, loud noises, changes in sleep patterns, hormones, and certain foods.

If you suspect your little one is having migraines, make an appointment with your pediatrician. Some pediatricians don't have a lot of experience treating pediatric migraines, so if your child isn't getting any relief, ask for a referral to a qualified professional.

Unfortunately, there are a limited number of prescription drugs approved or shown to be effective for child or adolescent migraineurs. Your doctor is most likely to recommend an over-the-counter medication. Acetaminophen (Tylenol®) and ibuprofen (Advil® or Motrin®) have both been shown to be relatively safe; there are more rigorous studies showing ibuprofen to be effective though acetaminophen seems to work faster when it does work. Nonsteroidal anti-inflammatory drugs (NSAIDs) are also sometimes used in treating migraines in children. If your doctor does prescribe a drug for your child, the usual choice will be a triptan that can be swallowed or dissolves in the mouth; some may consider injectable or nasal sprays as well. Specialists will sometimes also write a prescription for something that addresses the upset stomach as well.

The help you give your child should certainly go beyond

doctor's visits and medication. Be understanding, sympathetic, and supportive. Make sure your child has a dark, quiet place to sleep when she's in pain. Work with your child on tracking headaches and adjusting the environment to avoid possible triggers. Try not to let your concern turn into overprotectiveness. Although sleepovers, soda, and playing games outside on a hot, sunny day can all be triggers for migraine attacks, we don't advocate keeping a child from doing these things. Instead, try helping them track possible connections between triggers and headaches, and if they are old enough to understand, let them make their own decisions. Particularly in the case of adolescents, power struggles about diet and activities are rarely worthwhile. Instead, we find it is best to err on the side of letting the child live as normal a life as possible.

Children with migraines may occasionally miss school because of headaches, but if that turns into a regular occurrence, we recommend expert help. Repeated school absences not only impair academic progress but also prevent normal social activities and development. Work closely with school officials and nurses to keep children in school whenever possible. Sometimes this can mean going to the nurse's office for treatment rather than leaving school, or ensuring that a child who's had a morning headache that is now better goes to school in the afternoon.

You can take heart in knowing that some recent studies have found a number of children or adolescents with migraines either stop having headaches or develop less-severe ones as they reach adulthood.

Seniors

Shortly after Jean began receiving social security benefits, she experienced more good fortune. The frequency of her headaches—which had plagued her since her early thirties—began to diminish significantly. Not only that, they were less debilitating than in the past. This, she told her children, was finally something she could recommend about old age!

People over the age of sixty-five who have a history of migraines often report having fewer headaches that are less severe and come with fewer symptoms. Studies verify that, indeed, migraine prevalence decreases with age; only about 11 percent of older headache sufferers are diagnosed with migraines. Some even stop experiencing head pain per se but continue having visual auras or digestive issues. People who begin having migraines at a more advanced age often have an underlying medical issue and should see a doctor to pinpoint the cause.

One of the biggest challenges for older migraine sufferers is that they often have other health problems to contend with that involve taking medication on a regular basis. Some of these health issues, such as heart disease and stroke, narrow the choices of migraine medication owing to safety concerns. Certain medications can interfere with the efficacy of migraine meds. A health condition or medication may also be the source of migraine pain.

Another challenge for older migraine sufferers is finding the right treatment. Digestive, liver, and kidney functions tend to slow down with advancing age, causing the drugs to stay in the body longer. This can result in a different response and increased side effects to many of the mainstay and OTC migraine medications. Triptans are not recommended for those with heart and circulation problems; NSAIDS elevate blood pressure and increase the risk of kidney failure; opioids (sometimes called "narcotics") cause constipation, inpair judgement and can be habit-forming. What choices are left for the senior with a pounding headache?

Acetaminophen (Tylenol® and many prescription drugs) is generally considered safe for occasional use, and in fact some older migraine sufferers can take triptans or ergots safely and without excessive side effects; however, they must be thoroughly screened to make sure there are no conflicts with existing health conditions or competing medications. In our practice, when preventive treatment is necessary, we try to choose a daily or frequent-use medication that might also carry other benefits, such as controlling blood pressure.

One challenge for doctors in evaluating older people with headaches is to distinguish dangerous versus benign causes. Dangerous causes of headaches that are more common in older people include things such as stroke, high blood pressure, and various types of cancer. Older people are also more prone to developing inflammation of the arteries in the head, a condition known as temporal arteritis. This can produce headaches and other problems, even blindness, so it is important to diagnose promptly. Once identified, it can be treated with steroids, and once treated, the chance of visual loss is greatly diminished.

Domestic and Childhood Abuse, Neglect, or Trauma Victims

We once treated the wife of a prominent community member who endured stubbornly persistent headaches for years. We will always regret not asking her sooner about her home life because it eventually came out that she was the victim of domestic abuse.

Of course, not everyone who has migraines has been

the victim of abuse; nor does every abuse victim suffer from migraines. However, numerous studies have demonstrated a clear link between both domestic and child abuse and an increased likelihood of later migraine. For example, one study of more than seventeen thousand adults found that those who reported "adverse childhood events" were two times more likely than average to experience frequent headache attacks in adulthood. Other investigations reported earlier onset of headaches in abuse survivors than the average population.

We felt it was important to mention this issue so you are neither surprised nor offended should your doctor begin questioning you about a history of abuse. A physician who asks such questions is simply being thorough in the analysis of your headaches and is wise enough to treat the whole person rather than just the migraine. If in fact you are an abuse survivor or are currently in an abusive relationship, we urge you to speak up. Your doctor can help. And remember, doctors are ethically bound to maintain your privacy, so you can trust that what you reveal remains between you and your physician if that's what you wish. If, however, a doctor believes that any children or elders in the home are being abused or are otherwise in danger, he or she is obligated to report this to authorities.

Migraines and Increased Health Risks

For those with migraines, it's bad enough to have to put up with the pain! It doesn't stop there, though. They might also have to contend with other health risks associated with migraines, such as an increased chance of having a stroke or heart attack.

The idea that migraines might be linked somehow to vascular problems such as stroke and heart attack has been around for a long time, but the studies needed to evaluate this theory take a long time to do, so most of the strong evidence has come only in the last decade. One of the earliest studies to show a possible link was the Physicians' Health Study, which followed over twenty-two thousand doctors for a number of years. Those who reported having migraines were more apt to have a stroke, although not clearly more apt to have heart attacks. This early study was one of the first to suggest a connection between migraines and vascular problems, but it was not conclusive.

In the first place, the researchers didn't ask their subjects whether or not they had auras, so it wasn't possible to separate the risk for those who did have auras and those who didn't. In the second place, the diagnosis of migraines was never verified by a specialist.

However, other studies have also found an association

between migraines and these health risks, so now, after many decades of debate, most experts agree that people who have a history of migraine with aura have a slightly increased risk of stroke. This is true both when they are compared to people who do not have migraines at all, and when they are compared to people who have migraines without aura. The risk seems highest for women during their childbearing years, but also applies to men who have migraine with aura. Emerging evidence suggests that migraine with aura may be associated with an increased risk of cardiovascular disease later in life, too.

The reason for this link between migraine with aura and stroke and cardiac problems is not yet clear. It's possible that some of the things that happen in the brain to cause auras also cause small amounts of damage to the brain tissue or result in inflammation around blood vessels. Some studies have suggested that people with migraines and auras are more likely to have high blood pressure, diabetes, or other things that increase the chance of having heart disease or stroke as well.

We don't think this research is necessarily a cause for alarm. For one thing, the extra stroke or heart-attack risk an individual person carries because of migraine with aura is clearly small, especially in comparison to the health risks of things like smoking or high blood pressure. As of now, the bottom line is that people who have migraine with aura should be sure to do the routine things that can lower the risk of stroke and heart attack. You certainly shouldn't smoke, as this increases your risk of stroke and cardiovascular disease. You should exercise regularly and follow a heart-healthy diet to help maintain your weight, control your blood sugar, blood pressure, and cholesterol levels and to keep your cardiovascular system running as smoothly as possible.

If necessary, your doctor can prescribe medicines to help. Discuss with your doctor the possibility of taking a daily low-dose aspirin if you have a history of heart disease, stroke, or factors that increase your risk. Be sure to check with your doctor before starting aspirin. It may cause side effects, such as stomach ulcers. In the future, research will almost certainly help us identify which patients with migraines need to be especially vigilant about heart attack or stroke. Until then, there are good reasons for all of us to be vigilant about things that are known to affect these risks.

chapter 8

Migraine Medications

Throughout history, migraine sufferers have endured an odd array of alleged remedies. Ancient Romans zapped headache pain with a jolt from a black torpedo fish, or electric ray. In the thirteenth century, Europeans tried rub-on potions of vinegar. In 1660, a gruesome procedure dating back to prehistoric times known as trepanation—which involved drilling holes in the skull—was used as a migraine treatment. Erasmus Darwin, Charles Darwin's grandfather, proposed yet another bizarre treatment: spinning the patient in a centrifuge to force the blood from the head to the feet.

As we fast-forward to the present, modern medicine uses two types of medication approaches to help manage headaches: abortive or immediate-relief drugs that stop or improve a headache in progress and are taken when a headache strikes, and preventive (or prophylactic) drugs that keep headaches from developing and are generally taken daily. When recommending medications, your physician will consider a range of factors, including the type, intensity, and frequency of your headaches, other health problems you have, other medications you take, and your response to previous headache drugs.

It may take some time and effort to identify the most effective drug, combination of drugs, or dose, but patience and persistence usually pay off. Let's review some of the most commonly used migraine drugs; getting educated about available medications can help you and your doctor communicate more effectively.

Over-the-Counter Medications

Headaches are frequently triggered by stress, fatigue, lack of sleep, or a missed meal. Some rest or a bite to eat, perhaps together with an over-the-counter (OTC) pain reliever, is often the first course of action migraineurs will try long before they seek out medical attention. However, if you need to take an OTC pain medicine more than a couple of times a week, then you're suffering from regular, rather than occasional, headaches, and should see your doctor. Also, talk to your doctor if OTC medications don't ease your pain. These medications are ineffective for many people with severe headaches.

The following commonly used pain relievers (analgesics) are available in pharmacies and supermarkets. Many headache formulas fall into one of the categories below; others combine these substances and sometimes other drugs as well. Excedrin® Migraine, for instance, includes acetaminophen, aspirin, and caffeine. Keep this important thought in mind: Just because it's an OTC doesn't mean it doesn't have potentially harmful side effects.

- **Acetaminophen.** Acetaminophen (Tylenol® and others) is a generally safe nonaspirin analgesic though we have not found it terribly effective as a headache medication, either for prevention or to stop a headache in progress. Also, doses above the recommended level can cause health problems, so it's essential to read the labels carefully and never go beyond the recommended dosage or frequency of usage. If you've been taking acetaminophen consistently over a period of time, discuss this with your doctor. Your doctor may want to check your liver function. If you drink alcohol on a regular basis, consult with your doctor before taking an acetaminophen-containing medication; this drug has been linked to potentially fatal liver damage when combined with alcohol.

- **NSAIDs.** Nonsteroidal anti-inflammatory drugs (NSAIDs) include aspirin (see below), ibuprofen (Advil®, Motrin®, others), naproxen sodium (Aleve®, Anaprox®), and ketoprofen (Actron®, Orudis®, others). There is some evidence that daily doses of NSAIDs can help prevent migraine headaches, but we more often use them as an abortive rather than a preventive therapy due to their long-term side effects, which are similar to those for aspirin.
- **Aspirin.** Aspirin quells pain and may prevent migraine headaches in some people when taken regularly. Results from the Physicians' Health Study suggest that aspirin users experienced roughly 20 percent fewer migraine headaches during the study than did those receiving a placebo. Although low-dose aspirin is considerably less effective than the standard migraine-headache-preventive medications, it might prove useful when used in combination with a preventive medication. Some migraine patients have other reasons to be on regular aspi-

rin therapy. For example, daily aspirin appears to reduce the risk of stroke in some people. However, a decision to use aspirin daily should be discussed with your doctor, even though it is an OTC med, because in addition to possible benefits, there are also possible harms. Long-term side effects can include kidney damage and gastrointestinal problems, such as stomach pain, heartburn, or nausea. Bleeding from the stomach can also occur, often in such minute quantities as to go unnoticed, but sometimes in large amounts that can be fatal. Smaller levels of bleeding may cause anemia—which, in turn, may aggravate headaches. Avoid aspirin if you have reflux, gastritis, or an ulcer.

- **Caffeine.** Of all the treatments used for migraines, caffeine is perhaps the most controversial. Some experts believe it is a demon that plays a big part in causing or aggravating headaches, while others believe it is a helpful management drug. The truth seems to lie somewhere in the middle and may be different for each person. Caffeine is contained in many drinks such as coffee, soda, and tea, but it is also an ingredient in some headache medicines. Evidence from the Frequent Headache Epidemiology Study suggests that caffeine from both diet

> and medications is associated with the development of chronic daily headache. Additionally, there is good scientific evidence that even people who are not prone to headaches can develop them if they regularly use large amounts of caffeine, then stop it abruptly. It makes sense that people who already have a headache problem might be even more sensitive to the effects of caffeine.

For these reasons, we think a cautious attitude toward caffeine is prudent, and we advise patients that the absolute best approach for someone with headaches is probably to avoid dietary caffeine; for those who aren't willing to give it up, we suggest a daily limit of no more than one to two cups of coffee (or the equivalent amount of caffeine in soda or other drinks).

We can't deny, though, that many people, through trial and error, have struck upon a way to treat their headaches with caffeine; they might, for instance, down an aspirin with a cup of coffee or soda to deal with an oncoming headache. Others rely on caffeine-containing OTCs such as Excedrin® Migraine. While these strategies can be effective to a point, problems occur when caffeine is used on a daily basis, and the user develops dependence. Once this happens, any attempt at withdrawal becomes another headache trigger.

In our practice, we recommend limiting this medicinal use of caffeine to no more than once or twice weekly. If intermittent medical and regular daily use of caffeine doesn't appear to be out of control, we still caution the patient to keep an eye out for a relationship between consumption and pain but don't usually recommend abstaining. When we have patients we feel are overusing caffeine, we often recommend they give it up completely so they can get off the caffeine roller coaster. If the patient decides to give up

Decongestants

Some people with migraines self-treat with over-the-counter decongestants because they mistakenly believe they are suffering from a sinus condition. In fact, though decongestants may initially offer some relief, they can often make your migraines worse; they often lead you to a dead end in treatment. In many cases, they work less well after a while, and people then take more, which can lead to overuse, rebound nasal congestion, and systemic side effects. You should only use decongestants for short-term purposes. If you're still having headaches, they aren't the answer. Discussing things with your doctor is a better strategy.

caffeine, we recommend a stepwise approach to minimize any withdrawal headaches. For example, someone who is drinking five cups of caffeinated coffee a day might cut down by half a cup every day and eventually start mixing half-regular and half-decaffeinated coffee.

Prescription Preventive Medications

Beta-Blockers

Beta-blockers (used to treat high blood pressure and angina) and tricyclic antidepressants can reduce the frequency of migraine headaches by about half in a sizable proportion of patients. They can also reduce the intensity and duration of the headaches. Two beta-blockers, propranolol and timolol, are approved by the U.S. Food and Drug Administration for the prevention of migraine. Beta blockers probably dampen migraines through their effects on the nervous and vascular systems, although this is not known for certain.

How effective beta-blockers are in preventing migraine headaches varies from person to person and sometimes depending upon which one is used, so if the first one doesn't work, it's often worth trying another. Side effects can include fatigue, dizziness, cold hands and feet, exercise intolerance, insomnia, shortness of breath, depression, and impotence. Some beta-blockers can worsen asthma or other chronic lung disorders. They also may cause dangerously slow heart rates in unusual circumstances. Beta-blockers may on occasion worsen heart failure, although they benefit most heart-failure patients. People with heart and lung conditions who are on beta-blockers should be closely monitored by a physician.

Tricyclic Antidepressants

Although tricyclics were originally used as a treatment for depression, they are now more commonly used to treat various types of pain, including headache. In most cases, the doses used for headache are too small to adequately treat depression, and the drugs are effective for headache and pain in patients who are not depressed. As with other migraine-preventive drugs, tricyclics reduce headaches by about 50 percent in roughly half of people who take them. They are not approved for migraine prevention by the U.S. Food and Drug Administration, but they are widely used for this purpose, and we believe that the scientific and clinical evidence in support of their use is strong. It's not clear how the tricyclics work, but it is possible that they relieve pain by increasing the availability of the neurotransmitters serotonin and norepinephrine, which not only affect mood but also act to reduce pain signals.

When taking a tricyclic, you probably won't notice any benefit in the first week or two, and you may not feel its full effects for several weeks. However, some sedative effects are common early in treatment, which is a bonus for the many people with migraines who also have difficulty sleeping. Although a tricyclic could potentially improve mood, the doses prescribed for headache prevention are much lower than those used in treating depression. Side effects can include dry mouth, blurred vision, dizziness, weight gain, constipation, and difficulty urinating. People with a history of glaucoma, heart disease, or an enlarged prostate should avoid these drugs.

Calcium-Channel Blockers

Like beta-blockers, calcium-channel blockers are often prescribed for people with high blood pressure or heart disease, as well as for migraine prevention. But these medications work in different ways. Calcium-channel blockers relax muscle cells in blood-vessel walls and prevent blood-vessel spasm, which is what first prompted scientists to investigate their value for migraine prevention. As it turns out, however, calcium-channel blockers are probably effective at preventing migraines not because they increase blood circulation but because they act directly on nerve cells and thwart inflammation.

Treatment usually begins with a low dose that's increased gradually. Despite their name, calcium-channel blockers don't interfere with the absorption of calcium; nor do they cause calcium loss in the bones. Instead, they prevent the transmission of electrical signals—including pain signals—in the brain by blocking the calcium-ion channels that must open before such signals pass from one cell to another. Side effects include fatigue, dizziness, constipation, and swelling of the feet. Calcium-channel blockers may not be the best choice for people with heart failure or heart rhythm abnormalities. As with the tricyclics, calcium-channel blockers are not FDA approved for migraine prevention, but there is modest evidence from scientific studies to suggest they are useful.

Anticonvulsants

Two anticonvulsant, or antiseizure, medications are among the few medications specifically approved by the Food and Drug Administration for migraine prevention. Others are used for migraine prevention even though they are not specifically FDA approved for this purpose. Although the mechanisms are not entirely clear, anticonvulsants appear to work by reducing the transmission or perception of pain signals in the brain. In clinical trials, about half of the users who took topiramate or divalproex experienced a 50 percent or greater reduction in migraine frequency. However, beta-blockers and tricyclics are often better tolerated, so they may be a good starting point for treatment. Side effects of anticonvulsant medications vary depending upon the drug but can include nausea, diarrhea, weakness, weight changes (either loss or gain), and tremors. Very rarely, one of these drugs can cause potentially fatal liver failure (divalproex) while another one (topiramate) increases the chance of developing kidney stones. Nor are these drugs routinely recommended for women who are pregnant or trying to become pregnant. In fact, divalproex sodium (Depakote®) is a known cause of the birth defect spina bifida and should be used with great caution in any woman who might become pregnant. The anticonvulsant topiramate has also been linked to birth defects.

Prescription Abortive Medications

Ergots

The first drugs specially designed to treat individual attacks of migraine, known as ergots, are powerful vasoconstrictors (that is, they shrink blood vessels), but it is not clear that this is how they help ease a migraine. In 1938, researchers discovered that ergotamine tartrate—a drug derived from a fungus that can affect grain crops in wet weather—could abort migraine attacks, which led to the development of other drugs in this class such as dihydroergotamine and methysergide. Though one of the oldest classes of migraine-treatment drugs, they are still widely used worldwide.

Ergotamine rectal suppositories may be useful for severe headaches because they're absorbed faster than ergots in traditional pill form and can be taken even when you are sick to your stomach or vomiting. But all forms of ergotamine, including rectal suppositories, tend to cause nausea and vomiting—not a good side effect when treating a disease where that is already a problem. Apart from being unpleasant, an upset stomach hinders the absorption of medications. Antinausea drugs can be used, or you might try ergot drugs that are less likely to cause nausea, such as dihydroergotamine. Dihydroergotamine is now available in a nasal spray version; although easy to administer, in our experience it has proved much less effective than the suppositories, perhaps because the tissue lining the nose doesn't absorb medication very well. In contrast, lung tissue takes up drugs very effectively, which is why researchers are working to develop an inhaled ergot-based drug.

Botox®

Botulism is a rare but serious paralytic illness caused by a nerve toxin produced by the bacterium *Clostridium botulinum*. People usually contract botulism after eating contaminated food. Because botulinum toxin binds to nerve endings, essentially paralyzing motor nerves, physicians have used small doses of purified botulinum toxins, including onabotulinum toxin Type A (Botox®) to treat conditions caused by involuntary muscle spasms, such as writer's cramp and torticollis (limited neck motion or "wryneck"). In the 1990s, cosmetic surgeons began injecting it to smooth wrinkles and furrowed brows. Reports followed that people receiving Botox® for wrinkles on the forehead and between the eyes also coincidentally enjoyed improvements in migraine headaches.

Botox® (onabotulinum toxin Type A) was recently approved by the FDA for the treatment of chronic migraine (headaches fifteen or more days per month that last at least four hours), on the basis of two studies. However, a puzzling fact is that about half a dozen randomized double-blind placebo-controlled clinical studies—the gold standard in research—did not show a benefit of Botox® in treating episodic migraine. The reason for this is unclear–perhaps dosages weren't high

> enough or perhaps the medication only works on mechanisms that come into play once headaches are chronic—but from a clinical point of view we find that many patients with frequent, chronic headaches do report benefit from Botox® injections.
>
> Since FDA approval, some insurance carriers now cover the cost of injections while others have been slower to approve usage. In our own practice we have found that it can be effective though it may not work immediately, and it typically turns down the volume on headaches rather than banishing them completely. The protocol for headache injections is not the same as for cosmetic use, so it's important to have the drug administered by a trained specialist. Frequency of injection is typically once every three months though some of our patients are able to stretch this out. We find there is a very low dropout rate with this treatment; once patients find relief with this drug, they tend to stick with it.

Today, doctors are less likely to prescribe ergot-based drugs because some of them affect blood vessels throughout the body and therefore cause more side effects than newer medications, such as the triptans. Ergots may take longer to work than newer drugs; however, their beneficial effects last longer, so users are less likely to suffer a headache recurrence. Another reason that ergots have fallen out of favor is that many of them are not well absorbed when taken in pill form. New formulations of ergots such as better nasal sprays or inhalers may change that. One of the ergot drugs, dihydroergotamine, is highly effective when given intravenously, and it is one of our favorite emergency-department or in-hospital treatments for headache.

Triptans

Drug developers created triptan drugs in an effort to make a "cleaner" drug that worked on the same targets as traditional ergot drugs; that is, a medication that worked similarly but caused fewer side effects. These drugs relieve pain with far less nausea than most ergots, and if given as an injection, may begin to work within ten minutes. A sizable proportion of patients will experience complete or near-complete headache relief within one to two hours. Experts are not certain how triptans work to relieve migraine pain; theories include a decrease in inflammation around the blood vessels in the lining of the brain as well as constriction of blood vessels.

Doctors stress the importance of taking any oral migraine drug as soon as possible after your symptoms begin because as the headache progresses, a migraine can slow down gastrointestinal functioning, and the medications aren't absorbed as well. Several of the triptans are considerably slower to start working, but for many patients they may have fewer side effects, and their manufacturers claim they might be more effective in preventing the headache's return within twenty-four hours. That is a controversial claim, but these "gentler" triptans may be a good choice for patients whose headaches come on slowly and are mild but long-lasting. In nasal-spray form, some triptans can cut the time it takes for the medication to work by ten minutes or more, making them a good choice for more intense or faster-developing migraine headaches; on the other hand, some of the medication drips down the throat and can cause a bitter taste. For very-rapid-onset headaches, or those where nausea and vomiting occur early, there is nothing faster than an injectable triptan, which can provide relief in as little as fifteen minutes. Only sumatriptan comes in an injectable form, and it is available in a self-injector kit that is quite easy to use. The medication is deposited by a short needle just under the skin (subcutaneous injection because a deep muscle injection is not necessary). For patients who are afraid of needles, a needleless injection is available that uses a blast of air to create a hole in the skin through which the medicine then passes. Manufacturers are also working to develop a patch form of sumatriptan that will be absorbed through the skin.

If one triptan doesn't work, another often will. If a first dose of triptan doesn't work or (more likely) if it gives relief but the headache comes back, we recommend redosing with the same drug in accordance with the instructions on your prescription. If your headache still isn't completely relieved, you might consider taking aspirin or another NSAID along with the triptan. This combination strategy should, of course, be discussed with your doctor. When taking triptans, you may experience some mild side effects. All triptans can cause a temporary tingling in your fingers or tightness in your throat, while the nasal-spray or orally dissolving tablets can leave a bad taste in your mouth. The injectable form of sumatriptan, the only triptan that comes as an injection, tends to cause more intense side effects. On the other hand, triptans don't cause the nausea and vomiting common to the ergots; in fact, studies show they often relieve those symptoms.

Though certainly a mainstay migraine drug, many triptans are expensive. However, sumatriptan is now available in generic forms and can cost just a few dollars per pill. You can shop around and sometimes get your triptan prescription for less. And, although they can be effective much of the time, headaches often return within twenty-four hours. Depending on the dose, you will usually be able to take the same triptan again during a given twenty-four-hour period, but we don't recommend taking a different triptan or a similarly working ergot medicine to treat the same attack. Because triptans and ergots narrow blood vessels, taking them at the same time could lead to a heart attack. Not surprisingly, people with heart disease or uncontrolled high blood pressure shouldn't take these medications at all. Serious, life-threatening reactions to triptans are rare but do occur. Almost all of the reported cases have occurred in people who were known to have preexisting heart problems.

How much medicine is too much?

In general, we discourage patients from taking any medicine to treat individual attacks of headache more than two or three days a week. There are a number of reasons to avoid daily or near-daily use of triptans or any other medicine intended to treat individual attacks of headache. These drugs are meant to be used intermittently.

Depending upon the drug, daily use can increase the risk of side effects to unacceptable levels. For example, daily use of drugs such as ibuprofen or naproxen can cause stomach bleeding. Excessive use of acetaminophen can increase the chance of liver problems. Triptans affect blood vessels, and the effects of daily use on the risk of stroke or heart attack have not been carefully studied. Although they tend to hone in on cranial blood vessels, the triptans also manage to find receptors on the coronary arteries and, very occasionally, can cause chest pain that resembles angina. Yet large studies haven't shown an increase in the number of strokes or heart attacks among people taking triptans as prescribed, so the worry at this point is strictly theoretical.

The main reason we discourage use of these medicines more than two or three days a week is to minimize the chance the medication overuse headache (MOH) will arise. For complex reasons, many medicines used to treat individual headaches can actually make headaches worse—more frequent and more severe—if they are taken too often. The frequency of use needed to cause MOH probably differs from person to person and also may depend on the drug or drugs that are being used. However, most experts feel that MOH is unlikely to occur if use is limited to two or three days a week.

So if you're having migraines so often that you're taking sumatriptan or other drugs to treat individual headaches more than two or three days a week, it's probably time to take steps to prevent the headaches rather than just treating them when they occur.

Other Drugs

Prescription Painkillers

Prescription painkillers are more powerful than their OTC equivalents, and prescription-strength doses of NSAIDs can be very helpful for some patients. For example, an NSAID called indomethacin sometimes seems to work more effectively for certain types of headaches than other drugs in the class. It is available only by prescription, as an oral pill or as a 50 mg rectal suppository. We find that the suppository formulation of the drug works very quickly and can be used even by patients who are vomiting. This makes it very useful as a "rescue" treatment for bad migraine attacks. It sometimes keeps patients from having to go to the emergency room.

Combination prescription painkillers that contain the barbiturate butalbital (brand names Fiorinal®, Esgic®, Fioricet®) were once the most commonly used prescription drugs for migraines and other headaches. They have fallen out of favor for a number of reasons. In our experience, these drugs rarely relieve severe migraine pain. They also are very prone to be overused, and barbiturates taken regularly can be highly habit-forming.

Some prescription analgesics contain opioids. Opioids, such as codeine and morphine, are sometimes indispensable medications, but they have a limited role in the treatment of headache. People who regularly use opioids run the risk of developing a tolerance to them and, in some cases, becoming addicted. Tolerance means they need higher and higher doses to relieve the pain, and they develop withdrawal symptoms when they stop taking the medication. Also, most opioids impair judgment and driving ability and interfere with the ability to participate in everyday activities. In contrast, triptans and ergots usually do not cause significant problems with concentration or thinking.

If we use opioid or barbiturate combination medicines at all, we ordinarily consider them a "rescue drug"; when you have a severe headache and need something to make you feel better, this is a last-ditch effort to get things under control. The Frequent Headache Epidemiology Study identified a higher risk of progression to chronic daily headache in headache sufferers who used these drugs regularly. For this and other reasons, these are not drugs to be used as a first line of defense, and they should not be relied upon. If they are used, we find it helpful to have the patient agree on a limited number per month, and we are strict in sticking to this limit. This means the patient will have to pick and choose when and how to use the medication. While this may seem unkind, in the long run a careful limit like this will prevent the development of more serious problems.

Antinausea Medications

Migraine attacks often activate the autonomic nervous system, which is probably best known for its role in the "fight or flight" response. This affects the stomach and intestines, as well as other parts of the body. As a result, nausea and vomiting often accompany migraine headaches, which prevent you from keeping down your medications. Even when vomiting does not occur, the stomach takes longer to empty into the intestines once the sympathetic nervous system is activated—which can impair the absorption of oral medications.

To prevent vomiting, your doctor may recommend taking an additional prescription antinausea medication. Some suppress nausea and—because they have sedative effects—also help you sleep. Others help empty the stomach, thereby improving the absorption of oral headache medications. Some also counter the effects of a neurotransmitter known as dopamine, which may play a role in migraine attacks that is separate from nausea. In short, there are many reasons why these drugs can be very useful in the treatment of migraines. Many people find it particularly effective to take antinausea medication at the first hint of a migraine, then, about fifteen minutes later, to take the first dose of headache medication. Virtually all the antinausea drugs are available in several forms. If you can't take them by mouth, you can try rectal suppositories or, in extreme cases, injections.

New Drugs

Unfortunately, not all of the migraine mainstays work for everyone. This is why new drugs are constantly being tested and approved.

- **CGRP Receptor Antagonists.** One of the potential new migraine-abortive drugs belongs to a new class of medications known as CGRP receptor antagonists. CGRP is a chemical released from nerve endings that causes vasodilation as part of inflammation. A pill version of a drug that blocks CGRP has proven effective at quelling migraines within two hours in about two-thirds of people, according to one preliminary study. Unfortunately, this drug has failed to receive FDA approval because of the need to do more studies to evaluate possible side effects.
- **Inhaled DHE.** The lungs provide an excellent route to absorb medication quickly. Early tests of a special inhaled form of DHE found that the treatment curbs migraine pain in ten minutes. Called Tempo® Migraine, the drug also eased patients' nausea and sensitivity to sound and light. Additional testing in adults with asthma suggests that

they tolerate the drug well, despite their compromised lung function.

- **Memantine.** This is a receptor (NMDA receptor) blocker medication used to treat memory disorders but it has shown some benefit in small studies and case reports against pain and migraine, including possibly migraine-related aura symptoms. GI side effects are possible, and it can be difficult to obtain insurance approval to cover the cost of the prescription. It remains unclear if this will become a commonly used or FDA-approved headache therapy.
- **Doxycycline.** Headache specialists have all experienced the surprise of the unexpected benefit of a medication improving someone's headache situation when it was given for another reason. It's also a pleasant surprise for the patients. Doxycycline, a common antibiotic, is one such medication. Case reports suggest benefit from doxycycline in the treatment of some types of headache, especially an unusual pattern termed "new daily persistent headache." We have noted anecdotal benefit in an occasional patient as well. How it works is unclear though the medication functions as more than an

antibiotic and may inhibit inflammation. A detailed "At-a-Glance Resources and References" list of migraine medications is included in chapter 14.

Medication Overuse and Chronic Headaches

Be aware that transformation of an intermittent headache pattern to a daily headache often results from the overuse of OTC or prescription pain relievers. In other words, taking too much over-the-counter pain medication is actually a recipe for making your headaches worse! This phenomenon is sometimes referred to as *medication-induced headache* or *drug-rebound headache.* Some experts believe that any type of headache medication, when overused, can lead to chronic daily headache, although, confusingly, aspirin and ibuprofen taken on a daily basis are associated with a decreased risk of daily headache. In any case, there is general agreement that the drugs most often to blame for medication-overuse headaches are those that contain caffeine, which is a potent vasoconstrictor; that is, it tightens up the blood vessels. Medications containing butalbital and opioids may also be subject to overuse.

As many as 80 percent of chronic-daily-headache sufferers report excessive past use of analgesics, vasoconstrictors, or both. It is not always clear that the medications are responsible for the frequent headaches; in fact, it might work the other way. In other words, people might take medication excessively because they have so many headaches. In our experience, though, overuse of medications meant to treat individual headaches does seem to play a role in many complicated headache problems. We find that many patients improve when the drugs are withdrawn, and in any case, there are usually other medical reasons to decrease the use of these medicines. It is not clear how medication overuse makes headaches worse in some people. Researchers suspect that continued, regular use of some analgesics interferes with the body's natural painkilling system. Because analgesics mask symptoms, whatever is causing the pain may worsen. As the pain becomes more intense, analgesics are less able to control it. Or regular exposure to these drugs may change the way that the central nervous system responds to pain. Vasoconstrictors, on the other hand, may cause rebound vasodilation—and thereby possibly trigger a headache—when their effects wear off.

Because overuse of analgesics and vasoconstrictors can induce chronic daily headache, your doctor will ask you what type of medications you take and how often you take them. The doctor will also ask about your symptoms. People with medication-induced chronic daily headache may experience severe pain upon awakening, which then lessens as the day goes on—the exact reverse of the pattern most often seen in chronic daily headache. Such severe morning headaches probably result because any medication taken during the day has worn off during the night. The pain then subsides during the day as additional medication is taken. Additionally, people with medication-induced chronic daily headache sometimes report that they tried to stop the medication—and indeed went without it for a few days or a week—only to notice that their headaches got much worse. Such withdrawal headaches are typical of medication withdrawal and can last for several weeks, after which it can take weeks or months for the headache problem to subside. It is important to understand that headaches may first get worse, and only gradually get better, when overused medications are withdrawn.

When chronic daily headache results from overuse of painkillers, the first line of therapy is to stop taking those medications. Though practices do vary, in many cases, it's best to stop taking them at once, but the exact withdrawal strategy will depend on the type of medications you are taking and the types of symptoms you experience during withdrawal. In most cases, withdrawal from analgesic or vasoconstrictor dependency can be done on an outpatient basis.

If you are not able to tolerate the headache pain that occurs once medications are stopped, or if you experience nausea, vomiting, and muscle tightness in the neck and shoulder areas, your doctor may be able to provide other medications to ease the withdrawal process. If you have been taking significant amounts of medications containing opioids or barbiturates, the withdrawal process is likely to be more difficult, as these medications can cause a physical dependency. With barbiturates, for instance, it's best to gradually taper the medications to prevent seizures. Likewise, withdrawal from opioid dependency requires close medical supervision. In cases of extreme opioid or barbiturate dependency, you may even need to be hospitalized briefly.

chapter 9

Complementary, Alternative, and Integrative Treatments

When Heather came into our office, the first thing she told us is that she'd tried many headache remedies before but none had worked. When we asked her for specifics, she pulled out a plastic bag and dumped the contents onto the exam table. Out fell a large tube that looked like an oversized ChapStick®, a jar of cream, and a vial of clear liquid. The tube, she explained, was rubbed across the forehead over and over again so that menthol and herbs could be absorbed through the skin; the cream was massaged into the shoulders and under the neck; and the vial contained a solution of a highly diluted herbal remedy for her to splash onto her neck and face.

Heather said headaches were interfering with her life

several days a month but she was wary of taking medications because she was concerned about side effects and long-term effects. So, like millions of other Americans who suffer from all types of medical conditions, she'd decided to explore nontraditional treatments first.

Like Heather, many people who explore these options to cure or mitigate their migraines are hoping to avoid medication side effects, or they innately prefer a "natural" approach. Others are perfectly willing to take medication but haven't found one that works, or they're interested in trying these treatments in addition to taking prescription and OTC medications. Some avoid medication altogether due to religious or cultural beliefs or want to try something different because they've read about it on the Internet or have seen it advertised on TV.

Whatever the reasons, we certainly support the idea of trying all legitimate options to help ease headache pain. In this chapter, we help you sort through the myriad of nonmedical treatments by giving you the latest scientific and clinical information on which to base your decisions. This is sometimes easier said than done because many nontraditional treatments are not easily studied using typical scientific methods.

One of the biggest problems in assessing these treatments is that a patient's belief that a treatment might work may influence what happens when they try it. It's been well established that patients who have a strong prior faith in a particular treatment are indeed more likely to experience improvement with that treatment. This is often called a placebo response or placebo effect, but we prefer to refer to it as a "nonspecific" response because it's not related to the specific medicine or treatment being used, but rather to the patient's belief in what will happen. Interestingly, the opposite reaction can and does occur: Patients who have a strong prior belief that a medicine will be harmful or poorly tolerated are more likely to experience side effects or worsening when they take it. This is sometimes called a "nocebo" response. We think both responses illustrate the powerful influence of the mind on what happens in the body.

In testing medications, scientists need to separate nonspecific effects from benefits that are truly a direct cause of the treatment. They often compare how people who get the actual treatment do versus those who get a placebo or sham treatment; in the case of medicines, they often use a pill that looks like the real thing but doesn't contain its active ingredients. Typically, neither study patients nor researchers know which patients are actually receiving the real treatment versus a placebo. This helps keep prior knowledge and personal prejudices from influencing the results. Often, this is not possible with other types of therapies; it's pretty hard to disguise an acupuncture needle or hide a massage therapist!

Also, because many nontraditional treatments are not subject to regulation by the Food and Drug Administration, their manufacturers may not be required to do the kind of rigorous testing that is necessary for prescription treatments. For this reason, many study results looking at treatment alternatives aren't reliable, are difficult to reproduce, or the investigations don't last long enough to provide meaningful feedback. It's also the case that sometimes a procedure or therapy will work for one particular individual but not most other people.

Getting the Definitions Straight

Before we begin the discussion of migraine treatments that don't involve medication, it's important to understand some definitions. You will hear three different terms bandied about by health practitioners, patients, and others: *complementary, alternative,* and *integrative.* They are often used interchangeably, but they are not interchangeable. *Complementary medicine* refers to any treatment used in conjunction with conventional medicine; *alternative medicine* refers to any treatment used in place of conventional medicine; and *integrative medicine* refers to any treatment that seeks to combine the best of mainstream medical therapies and complementary and alternative (CAM) therapies. A treatment is typically put into a category depending upon how it's used. Many treatments can be used in a variety of ways and so can fall into more than one of the nonmedication categories. For instance, you might try a treatment as an alternative to medication at first but find it to be even more useful when combined with medications or other therapies. While many things that aren't a medicine or chemical have the potential to be useful in some way, there are also many dead ends and snake oils that will only waste your time and money.

Manual Therapy

Manual therapy refer to any therapy where the practitioner uses his or her hands to "manipulate" the muscles or other aspect of the body. The most popular manual therapies include physical therapy, massage, chiropractic, and trigger-point therapy. Based on patient reports and some small studies, physical therapy or massage may offer the most benefit, perhaps because they help to relax muscles.

- **Physical Therapy.** Physical therapists use techniques aimed at stretching muscles, improving posture, and increasing muscle strength. They also work on improving mobility in joints and try to address muscle imbalance or poor posture that may contribute to headaches. Physical therapists may also help patients develop a home exercise program.
- **Massage.** Massage therapists believe massage techniques may stimulate alternative sensory pathways and increase blood and lymphatic flow. How that might help headache isn't clear, but it's unlikely to be harmful, and many patients find it useful. There are varied massage techniques, so if this form of treatment appeals to you, it may be helpful to try out a few to see which, if any, are effective for you. Swedish massage, for example, involves long, smooth strokes, kneading, and circular movements on the superficial layers of muscle using massage lotion or oil. Shiatsu is a Japanese technique that uses localized finger pressure in a rhythmic sequence on "meridians" or predetermined points on the body. You should also be aware that massage techniques involving strong tapping or vibration, especially when done at or near the neck, have actually been known to make matters worse. We also hear from

patients who have significant sensitivity of the head and neck area so that any form of vigorous massage or other physical techniques can aggravate headaches; they may benefit from gentler forms of massage. Whatever the technique, it's best delivered by a trained and licensed massage therapist or physical therapist; requirements for licensure vary from state to state.

- **Chiropractic.** Chiropractors purport to help ease migraines through a combination of massage, spinal manipulation, and periodic adjustment of joints and soft tissue. While anecdotally many patients report no change in the frequency or severity of migraines after a chiropractic adjustment, a few studies have found it can offer some relief some of the time. Bear in mind, however, that it's difficult with this form of treatment to separate nonspecific from specific benefits. One thing we worry about with chiropractic treatment is the fact that it's often open-ended, so patients are tied to their chiropractic appointments indefinitely. Many patients keep regular appointments for years, which can be costly and time-consuming. We also feel concerned about a chiropractic technique known as high-velocity spinal manipulation. It should be avoided completely in the neck because it's been shown to cause damage and obstruct the large arteries that supply blood to the brain and has been associated with a risk of stroke. Since, overall, we don't think there is strong scientific evidence of benefit from chiropractic treatment for headaches, and given the small but serious risks associated with this treatment, we don't recommend it.

Electrical Approaches

The most common electrical technique we see used by our patients is transcutaneous electrical nerve stimulation (TENS). Other more involved, expensive, and less-frequently-employed procedures include magnetic stimulation, deep brain stimulation, and vagus nerve stimulation.

- **TENS.** A few small studies have shown that sending a very mild electrical sensation across the skin in TENS might reduce the frequency of migraines. Some practitioners suggest it's most effective when it's used in combination with medication, massage, and other traditional and CAM techniques, but we'd like to see more research confirming this before we'd consider recommending it routinely.

- **Implanted Occipital Nerve Stimulator.** The occipital nerve runs along the back of the head on either side, converging with the trigeminal nerve in the upper spinal cord. An occipital nerve stimulator consists of a pacemaker-like device connected to electrodes placed at the back of the head just under the skin. The electric current passing through these electrodes is thought to dampen activity in the trigeminal nerve, curbing migraine pain. This invasive treatment may only be appropriate as a preventive for people with chronic migraine who don't get relief from medications. At present we do not feel there is enough information to recommend this treatment to patients.
- **Transcranial Magnetic Stimulation.** We think the research is "suggestive" for transcranial magnetic stimulation. One company is working on developing a portable device that looks something like a small hairdryer and generates a focused, single magnetic pulse when applied over the scalp, which induces a mild electric current in the back of the brain. Some physicians and migraine experts believe this targeted signal might short-circuit the

hyperexcitability in areas of the brain associated with migraines. While an intriguing idea, magnetic stimulation is in the early phases of testing and, except in the context of a research study, it's not available for the average migraine patient.

- **Vagus Nerve Stimulation** (which requires a surgical procedure to place a wire that targets electrical impulses to the large vagus nerve in the neck) may also hold promise, but this is theoretical, and we need to see more scientific data before we can recommend headache-relief techniques that fall within this category.
- **Deep Brain Stimulation.** Originally used to treat depression, deep brain stimulation is under investigation to treat severe cases of cluster headache. This makes a certain amount of sense to us based on evidence that cluster originates in the brain. With deep brain stimulation, a medical device that essentially acts as a brain pacemaker is implanted in the head to send regular electrical impulses to specific parts of the brain. It seems quite helpful for some patients, but serious side effects have occurred, mainly complications such as infection, bleeding, or death, related to the surgical procedure to place the wire leads, so it is unlikely ever to be considered a first-line treatment. Might this

someday be tried for treatment-resistant migraine? Perhaps, but not for years to come.

Acupuncture

This is one of the most common treatments our patients try either before they come to see us or during the tenure of their medical treatment. It involves placing and manipulating long, thin needles into specific meridian points along the body that correspond to ancient Chinese astrological calculations; some practitioners also use traditional massage; a form of Chinese massage called Tui na, stimulate pressure points, or use herbal medicines and incense in conjunction with needles. Even though the results from scientific studies of acupuncture are mixed, in our experience some patients have reported dramatic improvements in their migraines from acupuncture. Why would this be so? We believe at least some of the benefit is likely to be nonspecific and also may relate to the therapeutic effects of one-on-one, individualized attention given by practitioners. Remember, a placebo response illustrates the powerful effect of the mind on the body. In the case of migraine, this relief in pain is just as "real" as the relief that comes from any traditional medicine. Although some patients and doctors look down their noses at treatments that might work because of placebo effects, we think there's great potential benefit in harnessing this "power of the mind." (In the next chapter, we'll discuss how methods like biofeedback, assisted relaxation, and meditation also take advantage of this mind-body connection.)

In acupressure, which is like a cross between acupuncture and massage, the therapist uses fingers and palms rather than needles to work meridian points. Like acupuncture, when it's used for migraine relief, the therapist will mainly focus work on the head, neck, and shoulders during treatment. Once again, some patients do anecdotally report some relief after a session. Unfortunately, we haven't seen these results backed up by any reliable, well-conducted studies.

Since so many of our patients say that acupuncture and acupressure have helped them, we usually don't try to convince them otherwise. In some cases, these treatments are covered by insurance, so, at the very worst, they get to relax on a treatment table for an hour—which in and of itself may be beneficial.

Energy Therapies

Homeopathy is part of a group of therapies that can be loosely termed "energy" therapies. Most are built upon the ancient Chinese belief that the physical body is a denser form of energy; tapping into these energy fields in various ways can change perception by the physical body. In the case of migraines, manipulating energy fields should theoretically help abate head pain. There are dozens of energy healing systems besides homeopathy; the ones most frequently mentioned by our patients include Reiki and Qigong.

- **Homeopathy.** The vial of diluted herbal remedy Heather brought with her during her initial visit was a sample of homeopathic medicine, a system of treatment where the individual is treated with a highly diluted substance with the goal of triggering the body's own innate healing powers. The belief of homeopathic practitioners is that "like cures like"; the diluted substance, when taken in large doses, will cause symptoms similar to the targeted disease, but in minute amounts, it will treat those symptoms. Most homeopathic substances in either liquid or pill form are diluted many hundreds of times over; tests in traditional labs often find no trace of the active substance whatsoever but believers are convinced that the water retains a "memory" of it.

  As you might expect, we remain skeptical of

homeopathic treatment; it's simply not compatible with modern scientific thinking. To date, there is little or no reliable evidence to show it offers any benefits to migraineurs at all—or any other health problem, for that matter—though you can never discount a placebo effect. Our concern with homeopathy is that people who go down this road waste their hard-earned money and a lot of time on something that has no chance of helping them.

- **Reiki and Qigong.** Reiki is a Japanese technique for stress reduction and relaxation administered by "laying on hands" to redirect the energy that flows through the patient's body/energy field. Practitioners believe that if your life-force energy is low or misdirected, you are more likely to get sick or suffer from maladies like migraines. Qigong (pronounced "chi gong") entails coordinating slow, fluid, dancelike movements with breathing to foster the flow of energy. Though there hasn't been much research looking at the efficacy of these methods for migraine sufferers, several major hospitals throughout the country offer these techniques to their patients with good if not scientifically verifiable outcomes. There has been no systematic scientific study of these techniques for headache, but they're

Plastic Surgery for Headache?—Look Younger and Be Headache-Free Too!

One group of surgeons recently published some stunning statistics about headache relief in patients who underwent standard facial plastic surgery: Writing in the *Plastic and Reconstructive Surgery Journal,* the surgeons claimed 80 percent of patients undergoing such procedures were headache-free at one year. Sound good? It does, but caution is warranted. This group, migraine experts believe, may not reflect the more typical migraine patient but rather a small subgroup of migraine sufferers with refractory headache related to specific, irritable scalp locations that have responded to prior treatment with Botox® (see chapter 8). Some experts surmise that one of the reasons for the striking results may be that the selection procedure has sorted out a small atypical group with a focal surface kind of pain. These people may experience headaches that otherwise still fit the definition of migraine but are not necessarily representative of the larger group of migraine patients. In this group, surgery might relieve pressure on small sensory nerves of the scalp and thus produce headache relief. It's an interesting possibility and a challenge to some of the current thinking among migraine specialists. However, whether this will become a widely used technique remains to be seen. In the meantime, it is worth remembering that large-scale, rigorous studies to prove the effectiveness and safety of this technique have not been performed.

unlikely to be harmful. As with any therapy that distracts patients from pain and provides a regular time to relax, these techniques may help the patient's overall well-being.

Supplements

Another common alternative to medications our patients frequently want to discuss is dietary supplements. There is a common misconception that since herbs, vitamins, and minerals are "natural," they're safer and have fewer side effects than migraine medications. This is not always the case. Also, since there is minimal government oversight for supplements, there's no guarantee that what's on the label is actually in the bottle. Look for products labeled "USP Verified," to ensure that what you're buying has been tested by the U.S. Pharmacopeia for purity and potency. Many supplements aren't cheap, so you want to get what you pay for.

If you're taking any sort of herbal remedy or supplement, it's very important to let your doctor know. Some supplements can be benign in and of themselves but cause serious reactions when combined with a medication or other supplements, or they may mitigate the effectiveness of your prescription medications. Don't exceed the recommended dosages either; too much of a good thing can sometimes cause unexpected and serious side effects.

- **Magnesium.** The mineral magnesium is frequently recommended to those who suffer from migraines, particularly women with menstrual migraines. There's some evidence to suggest that some migraineurs have low levels of magnesium in the brain; for those people, supplementing may lower the excitability of nerves in the brain as well as standardize the rhythm of the body's "biological clock" that controls sleep, temperature, blood pressure, hormone production, and other functions. Studies reviewing the use of this supplement to treat or prevent attacks have yielded mixed results. The typical recommended dosage is about 600 mg daily of a slow release form. Regular use is not without common side effects, such as gastrointestinal distress and diarrhea for some people. Besides supplements, consider getting your daily dose from foods such as fish, leafy green vegetables, nuts, and whole grains.
- **Riboflavin.** Also known as vitamin B2, this is another supplement commonly recommended to headache suffers. Foods high in riboflavin include

cheese, leafy green vegetables, meat, milk, yogurt, and enriched grains. It's thought to work by allowing cells to store energy without increasing the excitability of nerve cells. In several small trials, about half the people who took this supplement reported substantial improvements in the severity and frequency of their migraines but reported side effects including diarrhea, frequent urination, and bright yellow-orange urine. The recommended dosage for headaches is usually 400 mg/day in divided doses taken with food. Foods high in this vitamin include organ meats, almonds, bony fishes, eggs, and mushrooms.

- **Coenzyme Q10**. A substance naturally produced by the body's cells which is thought to diminish with age and with some health conditions such as migraines. Although many people now take CoQ10 for a variety of reasons, it's not clear whether or not supplementation works. Use remains controversial. However, in one small study, half the subjects taking 150 milligrams daily in supplement form reduced the number of days with migraines. Another study found similar results with 100 milligrams taken three times daily. It is generally free of significant side effects, but if you decide to try it, this is definitely one to check in with your doctor about. It can have interactions with various classes of drugs, including high blood pressure medications, blood thinners, and beta-blockers.

- **Fish Oil.** Fish oil is rich in omega-3 free fatty acids commonly found in fish, walnuts, flaxseed, and leafy green vegetables. People in Western countries often eat diets that are low in omega-3s. Omega-3 fatty acids may decrease migraine frequency, duration, and severity, perhaps because they have the potential to decrease inflammation and prevent blood clots. Some studies link platelet clumping to the migraine process, and a few standard migraine drugs (such as aspirin) decrease the tendency of platelets to aggregate. Studies showing the effectiveness of omega-3s to offer migraine relief have been disappointing. Many people report annoying side effects like fish breath and burping; more seriously, if you notice any bruising or bleeding while taking this supplement, talk to your doctor.
- **Herbal supplements.** Two common herbal migraine remedies are butterbur and feverfew. Both are flowering plants related to the common daisy and chrysanthemum respectively and thought to reduce inflammation, which in turn might reduce

the number and intensity of migraines. Both of these supplements have been studied scientifically although the trials for feverfew in particular were small and not especially rigorous; a recent summary of all of this research concluded that the evidence feverfew is helpful for migraine is not very strong. The evidence for butterbur is somewhat better but limited to just a few good-quality studies. Nonetheless, some patients report benefit with these supplements. With feverfew, patients who notice a benefit often report that it takes several weeks to occur and in the meantime, some develop mouth ulcers and stomach problems. If you're taking a blood thinner or have any history of bleeding problems, check with your doctor before taking this supplement; abrupt discontinuation of this supplement may actually increase your headaches, cause sleep problems, or make you feel irritable, so if you do decide to stop using it, be sure to wean yourself off gradually. We advise that pregnant and nursing women, young children, and those with liver or kidney disease should not use butterbur. And beware: If you have allergies to daisies, ragweed, marigolds, or chrysanthemums, you may also have allergies to these two supplements.

- **Melatonin.** The "sleep hormone" might theoretically influence migraine symptoms in a number of ways, from exerting a direct antiheadache effect to influencing headaches through its helpful effect on sleep. Its use in headache is based on evidence from a relatively small number of cases, but many headache specialists still mention it to their patients. The dose usually ranges from 3 to 6 mg nightly and higher in cluster-headache patients. It is more commonly associated with treatment of jet lag, however since these time shifts are often a trigger for headache, its use in migraine is not completely without logic. Plus, it appears to be essentially free of side effects.

As Seen on TV

It might be easy to laugh at people like Heather, who spend their money on herbal headache sticks and rub-on creams they've seen advertised on late-night TV alongside juicers and flimsy exercise machines, but as a migraine sufferer, you know how tempting it is to try *anything* when you're in the midst of a bad headache. It's truly unfortunate that marketers capitalize on people's pain and desperation, but since they do, the buyer must beware.

The products purchased by Heather are just a sampling of what's being hawked both on TV and on the Internet to people with migraines. The products range from the strange to the completely ridiculous. Many of them involve some form of cold therapy, which to our knowledge has never shown any promise for helping migraines, while some involve wearing magnets around the wrist to redirect the earth's magnetic waves—something we doubt is possible from something that is essentially a refrigerator magnet.

When it comes to migraine remedies that are not recommended by a health-care professional, it's truly buyer beware. We hate to see people waste their money and suffer needlessly chasing down phony cures when they have not had a chance to try remedies that have been proven effective.

chapter 10

Lifestyle Changes

The majority of approaches to managing migraines we've discussed thus far can be quite effective, but, to a large extent, they are passive, requiring you to take a drug or rely on a practitioner of some sort. Over the years, we've found that our patients who do best—even when they don't necessarily get immediate results—are the ones who feel empowered to take some control over their migraines.

This is the beauty of making simple lifestyle changes. Learning to manage key aspects of your everyday life may not only help you gain relief from migraines; it can also reassure you that you yourself hold the key to managing your own health. So many of our patients tell us that taking steps to become more self-reliant about their headaches provides relief in and of itself. And beyond migraine treatment, living a more sensible, healthier lifestyle is good for you in a myriad of other ways.

The lifestyle aspects we cover in this chapter are those we've observed to be the most helpful—and controllable—for our patients, and for which there is at least some scientific evidence that supports our clinical observations. They are: regular physical activity, adequate and regular sleep, and relaxation. We've also included a discussion about food. Although evidence is mixed about whether certain foods either trigger or relieve migraines (see chapter 3), many of our patients have a strong belief that food does have an effect on their headaches. Since this is the case, we often find it useful to work with them to identify their dietary culprits and heroes. As long as keeping a food diary and manipulating diet doesn't become a burden, there's probably no harm in exploring the connection between what you eat and how your head feels.

Exercise

Most headache specialists recommend that their patients exercise and increase their overall physical activity, but to date, the evidence that physical activity actually guards against migraine attacks is skimpy. A few studies have shown that taking regular exercise can reduce the severity, though not the number, of headaches. One such study was done by Austrian investigators; it found that after six weeks of twice-weekly workout sessions, their thirty female volunteers did indeed report their migraines were less intense, and they also felt less depressed. (Remember, many experts suspect that depression and migraines are linked.)

The majority of other investigations and case studies have concluded that exercise had no benefit whatsoever when it came to reducing migraines. However, anecdotally, a number of our patients have confided over the years that exercise seems to help reduce their migraines' frequency and severity. Many say they get the most-noticeable improvements when their workouts are hard-core and high-intensity. We haven't seen any literature to back up these claims but find them worth paying attention to since it's mentioned so often by patients. That said, some patients say that high-intensity exercise exacerbates their migraine problems, possibly due to dehydration or an increase in heart rate and blood pressure; but for the most part, people with migraines can exercise moderately without making matters worse. This is a case where individual responses likely make the difference.

We certainly encourage all of our patients to exercise on a regular basis. We believe that strengthening your heart and lungs and keeping your weight down can only work in your favor when trying to overcome any health issue, migraines included. Our recommendations of thirty minutes of physical activity most days of the week are in line with those of health groups such as the American Heart Association and the American College of Sports Medicine.

Sleep

Migraineurs commonly complain of poor, fragmented sleep and feeling unrefreshed when they wake. In fact, adults with severe headaches are at significantly higher risk of also suffering from sleep problems, when compared with the general population, regardless of specific headache type.

Most of us go through about six sleep cycles each night, with about four stages of sleep, plus rapid-eye-movement (REM) sleep. The third and fourth stages are the deepest stages of sleep and essential for the adequate production of the "feel good" neurotransmitters, serotonin and dopamine. Some people with migraines appear to suffer from lack of, or scrambled, REM sleep; this can trigger a migraine through effects on these brain chemicals as well as other factors.

Although many patients tell us that sleeping too much or too little can trigger a migraine, there is no absolute optimum amount of sleep we can recommend for migraine management. It's probably different for every individual though we suspect (and studies suggest) it's probably somewhere around eight hours for most people. Surprisingly, there are very few studies that have investigated whether or not getting better sleep can improve migraines. The few that have been done do indicate that making an effort to get better-quality sleep will be a helpful migraine-prevention strategy.

When assessing whether or not poor sleep could be contributing to your migraines, ask yourself: Do I have trouble getting to sleep? Do I frequently wake up several times during the night? Do I feel unrested in the morning? Am I often awakened by headaches in the middle of the night or have one upon waking?

If you answer yes to many of these questions, it surely can't hurt to try getting more and better-quality sleep to manage your headaches. Go to bed at the same time every night, at a time that allows for eight hours in bed. Eliminate TV watching, reading, or listening to music while in bed and establish a calming, relaxing routine at bedtime. Avoid caffeine, nicotine, alcohol, fluids, and eating in the last few hours before bedtime. Avoid daytime naps and get plenty of cardiovascular exercise, though not right before bedtime. If you snore, or if your partner tells you that you sometimes appear to stop breathing while sleeping, it's worth mentioning this to your doctor. You may have sleep apnea, a condition that is associated with headaches, particularly those that occur in the morning. Sleep apnea is diagnosed with a sleep study, in which you sleep in a laboratory while brain waves, breathing, and oxygen levels are monitored. If there is evidence of obstruction of your breathing and substantial drops in your nighttime oxygen level, it can be treated with a special nighttime breathing mask, or occasionally with surgery to improve airflow through the back of the throat.

Relaxation

One of the biggest advantages of relaxation techniques is that you can practice them almost anywhere and in any situation. So, if a migraine comes on, say in the middle of an important meeting, you can try and work through it using some simple skills. Most relaxation methods don't require special equipment or expert trainers although it's often helpful to have the support of an instructor or group to help master the basics. Some people also practice other mind/body strategies, such as yoga and tai chi, to augment their relaxation techniques.

There are many ways to get to an end result of a calmer body and mind, from straightforward breathing techniques to full yoga and meditation practice. Rather than choosing just one technique to elicit the relaxation response, consider sampling many until you find a combination that suits you. If your favorite fails to engage you sometimes, it's good to have a fallback plan. In fact, many people get the best results from combining several techniques.

Thus far, biofeedback and meditation are two of the most evidence-based relaxation techniques. That doesn't mean other schools of thought on relaxation aren't valuable for migraine relief, it just means they haven't been adequately studied yet.

Biofeedback

Biofeedback is a relaxation technique that helps you gain conscious control over body processes that are normally unconscious, such as blood pressure and the tension level in your muscles. By learning to control those functions, you may be able to improve your migraines as well as other health problems you're experiencing.

The evidence for biofeedback's providing a reprieve from migraines is stronger than just about any other non-drug technique; in studies where it's compared to standard medication such as a beta-blocker, benefits have been shown to be comparable, and when used in combination with medication, headache benefits are even greater.

Pediatric migraine sufferers in particular seem to gain value from this method, perhaps because they approach it with a sense of fun like they would a video game. For example, a recent report in the journal *Neurology* followed twenty preteens with migraines as they practiced age-appropriate biofeedback techniques three times a week (and whenever they had a headache) for two weeks. At the end of the evaluation period, the majority of the tweens reported marked differences in both severity and frequency of their headaches plus they missed fewer school days. More than 85 percent of parents said their kids were functioning better as the result of their training.

However, we don't want to leave you with the impression that biofeedback is some sort of quick-fix migraine cure. It requires motivation, time, effort, practice, and honest communication with your therapist for you to get meaningful results. To get the most from your sessions, your therapist should discuss your symptoms and expectations, medical history, current medications, and any other treatment you've tried in the past. You should review the results you hope to achieve and the results you can expect.

A typical session starts with the biofeedback practitioner pasting electronic sensors onto your body to detect changes in your pulse, skin temperature, muscle tone, brain-wave pattern, or some other physiological function. These changes trigger a signal: a sound, a flashing light, or a change in pattern on a video screen that tells you that the physiological change has occurred. Gradually, with the help of your biofeedback therapist, you can learn to alter the signal by taking conscious control of your body's automatic body functions. After a few sessions, many people are able to continue biofeedback on their own. The number of sessions you will need depends on how quickly you take to this method.

Biofeedback is generally a safe form of therapy. There are no state laws that regulate the training of biofeedback therapists, but many therapists voluntarily obtain a certificate from the Biofeedback Certification Institute of America (BCIA) as proof of their education, experience, and professionalism. Before you begin biofeedback therapy or any other form of alternative therapy, we suggest you check your therapist's credentials, experience, and certification. Some (though not many) insurance carriers cover part of the cost of biofeedback sessions. If you can't find a practitioner near you, consider buying a book or downloading a video to learn it on your own.

Meditation

The goal of meditation is to clear away the stress-inducing thoughts that crowd the mind. Practicing meditation can give you a sense of peace, improve your psychological balance, and enhance your overall health and sense of well-being.

A tremendous body of research connects regular meditation practice with diminished pain. Meditation appears to train the brain to be more present-focused and, therefore, to spend less time anticipating future negative events. Researchers have found that particular areas of the brain are less active as meditators anticipate pain; there is also some unusual activity in part of the prefrontal cortex, a brain region known to be involved in controlling attention and thought processes when potential threats are perceived. Further, regular meditation has been shown to alter the cerebral cortex over time, a change which has been associated with better pain tolerance. The more practice meditators have, the more effective pain management appears to be; however, some studies have noted improvements in as little as a few sessions.

In the few investigations that have been carried out, meditation and activities such as yoga that incorporate meditative skills seem to show specific promise in helping to reduce migraine pain. One Indian study provides a good illustration of this. The researchers had a group of subjects practice a yoga meditation for one hour a day, five days a week, for three months. Compared to subjects who were educated about other aspects of their lifestyle such as diet and exercise (but didn't necessarily follow through with these changes), the meditating subjects saw a significant reduction in both number and severity of migraine attacks. As a bonus, the meditators also reported significantly improved symptoms of anxiety, stress, and depression. These results fit with research using special scans that show brain activity during painful events. People who are distracted from pain (as might happen with meditation) have decreased activation in the parts of the brain that notice pain.

There are many different types of meditation, most of which originated in ancient religious and spiritual traditions, though meditation does not require a spiritual or religious aspect to be effective. Two of the main forms of meditation are *concentrative meditation*, which involves the silent repetition of a word, thought, or phrase, as you try to clear your mind of distracting thoughts; and *mindfulness meditation,* also known as Zen or insight meditation because it focuses on the here and now. During mindful meditation, you usually start by observing your breath, then turn your attention to the thoughts, feelings, and sensations you're experiencing, without judging or analyzing them.

You can practice these techniques in less formal ways to help bring mindfulness to your usual routines. Whether you are eating, showering, walking, driving, or playing with a child or grandchild, slow down as you go about each activity, bringing your full awareness to both the activity and your experience of it.

When You've Got One Minute to Relax

Place your hand just beneath your navel so you can feel the gentle rise and fall of your belly as you breathe. Breathe in slowly. Pause for a count of three. Breathe out. Pause for a count of three. Continue to breathe deeply for one minute, pausing for a count of three after each inhalation and exhalation. Or alternatively, while sitting comfortably, take a few slow deep breaths and quietly repeat to yourself "I am" as you breathe in and "at peace" as you breathe out. Repeat slowly two or three times. Then feel your entire body relax into the support of the chair.

Food

As we discussed in detail in chapter 3, many foods have been labeled migraine triggers, most commonly chocolate, aged cheeses, cured and processed meats, and foods containing the chemical MSG. Surprisingly, there's little actual evidence to support any specific foods as headache triggers yet we suspect that some people are indeed susceptible.

A common recommendation by many headache specialists—and from one migraneur to another—is to keep a detailed food diary to help pinpoint which foods may be causing problems. The idea is that once you identify a potential trigger, you can eliminate it from your diet and see if things get better. If the situation does in fact improve, you're on the right track. If not, you can continue tracking to try to get to the root of the problem.

For those who have taken the time to fill out a food diary, we always take the time to review it in detail with them. We provide several examples of food diaries in chapter 4 for those who want to try this exercise. However, for some, keeping track of their food for days on end can be tedious and actually add to the stress of migraines. Should you find this is the case for you, it's probably not worth the effort.

The most commonly reported dietary triggers are alcohol and skipped meals. In studies, skipped meals and fasting are reported by more than half of participants as a reliable migraine trigger. It's believed that going for as little as five hours without eating may alter brain chemicals, hormones, or the metabolic process in ways that promote headaches. One thing that is probably *not* playing a role here is blood-sugar levels. Although people commonly speak of having "low blood sugar" when they haven't eaten for a while, blood-sugar levels are tightly regulated by the body. In patients who do not have diabetes, it is uncommon for blood-sugar levels to fall dramatically. Instead, the changes we notice when we are hungry are likely due to other hormones and bodily changes that occur when we haven't eaten for a while. So, obviously, the overarching advice here is that a good way to avoid a thumping headache is to eat regular meals.

Another fairly reliable trigger is alcohol. For some, even a couple of sips of alcohol can bring on a headache within minutes. The cause of an immediate alcohol-triggered headache is probably vasodilation although the exact cause of hangover headaches that occur after substantial amounts of drinking is likely different and is still not completely understood. Suffice it to say that it is probably a wise move to avoid alcohol if you find that it consistently results in throbbing head pain. If you do drink, stay well hydrated and make sure to have some food in your stomach. And again, though often patients will report specific difficulty with wine, especially red wine, studies to date do not provide strong evidence that one sort of alcohol is more likely to cause a headache than any others. Nonetheless, if a particular sort of alcohol seems to be the culprit behind some of your headaches, it is best to avoid it. When they gain control of their underlying headache pattern, we find that patients occasionally report that they are able to add a small amount of alcohol back into their diet without adverse consequences. Always check with your doctor, though, to make sure alcohol in small amounts is compatible with the medications you are taking.

Finally, as we discussed at length in chapter 3, caffeine can be both a gift and a curse for migraine sufferers. On the one hand, some people find that caffeinated drinks help manage their migraines, probably owing to caffeine's mild pain-relieving properties, because it may constrict blood vessels or because it increases the absorption of other pain medications they've taken. On the other hand, caffeine can cause dehydration, which can lead to headaches and, once the stimulating effects of caffeine wear off, you can crash hard, especially if you haven't had anything to eat. Caffeine withdrawal, especially a cold-turkey withdrawal,

Could Wheat Be Your Problem?

People who have celiac disease have trouble digesting gluten-containing foods such as wheat, barley, rye, and, possibly, oats. Gluten can also be found in medicines, vitamins, and even the glue on stamps and envelopes. When those with the disease eat foods with gluten, their immune system responds by causing damage to the small intestine. Symptoms vary, but scientists are beginning to think it may cause headaches that can mimic migraines, or aggravate migraines in those who already have them. For example, one Italian study that followed ninety migraine sufferers determined that four had celiac disease and had those subjects follow a gluten-free diet for six months. During this time, one of the four patients had no migraine attacks, and the remaining three patients experienced an improvement in frequency, duration, and intensity of migraines.

Some evidence suggests that occasionally people can be sensitive to gluten but not have the immunologic or intestinal changes of celiac disease. This situation is referred to as gluten sensitivity or gluten intolerance. If gluten-containing foods pop up as a possible trigger on your food diary, it may be worth getting a simple blood test to determine whether you could have celiac disease. We've had patients who have tested negative for the condition yet still insisted that limiting their gluten intake made a big difference in migraine management. Of course, this could be a nonspecific or placebo effect (see chapter 9 for more details) but we rarely stop a patient from using a successful strategy unless we feel it's harmful.

can also result in intense headaches. Migraine-susceptible patients should seriously consider limiting their daily intake to less than 200 mg of caffeine a day, realizing that caffeine also is found in tea, cola, chocolate, and even some non-cola beverages. If you don't drink anything with caffeine already, we recommend you don't start.

chapter 11

Migraine Management

Family Matters

Nia comes from a close family. Perhaps too close. The first time she came into our office to talk about her recurring headaches, she brought her mother, husband, and two teenaged daughters in tow. When asked a question about her symptoms and headache patterns, one of Nia's loved ones was either quick to jump in with a response or corrected the response that Nia herself gave. After fifteen minutes of this, Nia's family was politely escorted to the waiting room for the rest of the visit.

This is something we headache specialists witness on a regular basis. The migraineur's family is so heavily invested in the person's suffering that much of the family dynamic is built around it. Everyone in the family seems to experience, if not the actual pain, then the "event" of the migraine.

Sometimes the opposite is true: Diane, another patient of ours, is a migraneur who got no sympathy or support from her family and had to go it alone. Having never experienced a headache, her husband, Dave, didn't take them seriously. He didn't feel that Diane's headaches were real and believed she used them as an excuse not to attend family functions or go to work. Often, he'd actively go out of his way to prevent her from coming in for treatment. Once he even went so far as to tear up her prescription. When we see this dynamic, we pay attention. At times, but not always, it can be a manifestation of an abusive relationship; we discuss the link between migraines and abuse in chapter 7.

Nia and Diane seem to have polar opposite family situations. Both of these scenarios add challenges to treatment and overall management because both make it more difficult for the headache-prone person to take control of the problem. If either is the case for you, it's worth considering how your home life could be affecting your migraines.

Migraines Take Their Toll

Even when family members are appropriately supportive, migraines can stress out relationships. Though few studies have examined the impact of migraines on the family, the ones that have, show it can wreak havoc. Half of people with migraines who live with someone believe their headaches make them more likely to argue with their partner—and nearly 30 percent of their partners agree. A significant number of people with migraines also report having a diminished ability to do household chores, avoid making plans for fear of canceling due to headache, and believe they would be better partners if they didn't have headaches.

A good percentage of people with migraines say headaches tend to place strain on relationships with their children, too. It's especially hard on young children, who may not fully understand what *mommy has a headache* means. Kids can sometimes find it difficult to accept that a parent may need the lights dimmed and the house quiet—and it may be a little frightening that someone they love and depend upon is sick.

The bottom line is that migraines steal away family time and disrupt the household. It may be uncomfortable for the person with the migraine to admit, but living with the migraine sufferer can be trying at times. That's why it's so important to spark an open and honest dialogue with your loved ones.

Making Them Understand

Start by asking your family members to be patient with you. Of course, you would prefer to help with homework or make sure the taxes get done on time, but sometimes the pain makes it impossible. Let them know you are doing the best you can and that when you are able, you will be there for them. Keep in mind that this may not be easy for some family members to process, especially young children and those who have never experienced any sort of chronic pain themselves.

If, like Diane, you have a nonbeliever in the family, consider taking the doubter along on a doctor's visit. When Dave came to one of Diane's appointments, it was a turning point in their relationship—and in her treatment. For the first time, he was enlightened about how migraines are not only real, they are more than simply bad headaches and, in fact, are a neurological disease. Hearing the doctor explain what Dave's wife was going through finally made Dave understand the terrible, throbbing pain she endured on a regular basis.

During this visit, we also recommended that Diane

share some informational resources with Dave and the rest of her family members so they could gain a better understanding of her migraines. If you flip to the Resources section, you'll find an abundant list of reliable resources to share with your family, most of which are accessible on the Internet. And, of course, you can always share the information in this book.

We've also noted that getting the family actively thinking about migraine management can be a valuable experience for everyone; but again, this is only true as long as they don't cross the line and become too invested. Set boundaries during headache times and ask them to accept your downtimes. Have your family help you work around your triggers. Let them know what you need—and then thank them for doing it. All of these simple communications go a long way toward making you feel loved and your loved ones feel proactive and compassionate. We consider that a win-win.

However, not everyone is as fortunate as Diane in getting loved ones to see the light. It's possible that, despite your best efforts, you may be stuck with a family member who refuses to be supportive or understanding or one who makes it worse because they won't back off from trying to fix your problems. This undoubtedly adds to your burden; but ultimately, the path of least resistance may simply be to accept this and find ways to live with their behavior. Sadly, sometimes it won't be win-win.

Migraines at Work

Your coworkers may like you, even respect and admire you, but they aren't married to you or related by DNA. Plus, you all have a job to do, and they expect you to pull your weight. This is why "I have another migraine" will not always be met with empathy in the workplace.

Migraine frequency tends to peak during prime working years, which leads to maximum cost for both the employee and employer. On the individual side, surveys and studies report that those with chronic migraines miss significantly more time at work thanks to headaches, and when they tried to work through the head pain, their productivity was reduced by more than 50 percent. The majority of economic burden realized by employers can be chalked up to lost productivity, a combination of costs attributable to absenteeism and to lost efficiency while on the job. One large financial services company reported losses of $21.5 million from migraine-related absenteeism and $24.5 million stemming from reduced on-the-job productivity.

Dealing with Migraines at Work

No one likes to miss work or turn in less than one's best effort. But if you suffer from migraines, you may find yourself in this position more often than you prefer. The wisest strategy is to be totally up-front with your superiors and coworkers.

Explain your situation, then respectfully yet firmly ask for their understanding—but be prepared to hear that not everyone will get it or will rally to your support. Our patient Olivia had a boss who was very impatient and negative about her migraine episodes—until he had one himself. Once he experienced the throbbing, unrelenting pain for himself, he quickly realized it wasn't Olivia's bid to dump her work onto her coworkers or leave early. He's now very sympathetic to her situation.

At the same time, you probably want to avoid the "over share." While most people are genuinely concerned about you and wish you well, they also don't want to hear your laundry list of complaints; nor do they want to do extra work to pick up your slack. Would you? You are going to be better off making sure everyone is aware of your migraines but keeping discussion about them to a minimum. Do the best job you can, avoid causing too much drama, and try to disrupt the flow of the workday as little as possible. And again, accept the fact that some of your coworkers, some of the time, may not be as understanding as you would like.

If you've got a particularly prickly boss, consider asking for a note from your doctor that explains the details of your condition. In larger companies, this can be filed with the medical, benefits, or human resources department. Having a letter in your file can smooth the process should there be a dispute about missed work, loss of productivity, or you need to apply for disability leave down the road. By the way, it is vitally important to discuss the level of disability you experience both at home and at work with your physician. Pain is subjective. This information has a powerful influence on physicians' perceptions of illness severity, treatment choice, and the need for follow-up.

Insurance Disputes

Insurance companies can be notoriously arbitrary about which migraine drugs they cover—and how they cover them. For example, some try to limit the amount of triptans you can be prescribed in a certain period of time and may imply that the Food and Drug Administration (FDA) sets such limits. In fact, the FDA has jurisdiction over the pharmaceutical industry—but not the insurance industry; therefore, any such implications are unfounded. If the issue is about generic versus brand medication, keep in mind that in most cases, generics should be just fine and may well be worth a try.

If you do dispute limitations of coverage, do some research so you know your facts. We find that it helps to remain persistent but polite. Check with your doctor's office to see if they are able to provide help; they can sometimes explain more effectively why you are being prescribed a certain treatment, which may influence your chances of getting coverage. Please bear in mind, though, that many office staffs are overworked and find that such advocacy takes up a fair amount of their time. Though they are often happy to fight for the patient, they have other responsibilities as well. Keep your workplace benefits department in the loop about any insurance coverage or claim disputes you may have, too. In many instances, they have more clout than you do to get things pushed through.

Taking Leave

Two federal programs, Social Security Disabilities Insurance (SSDI) and Supplemental Security Income (SSI), may allow you to take unpaid leave from your job if your migraines become too much to handle, especially if you work for a company that employs more than fifty people. Whether or not you are covered depends on your specific circumstances. The Family and Medical Leave Act (FMLA) grants employees a total of twelve weeks of unpaid leave during any twelve-month period for several reasons, among them when the employee is unable to work because of a serious health condition. Your medical, benefits, or human resources department should be able to provide you with all the information you need about FMLA, but if they are less than forthcoming, check with the U.S. Department of Labor (http://www.dol.gov/dol/topic/benefits-leave/fmla.htm).

Even if you are not eligible for FMLA, you may be covered for disability leave by other company policies or laws. More information about SSDI and SSI are available at your local Social Security Administration office.

Building a Support System

Support comes from many places. Besides your family and coworkers, you may find a helping hand from a friend, neighbor, clergy, support group, or perhaps even an online chat room. Having the right support is every bit as important as having the right medication. Without it, you can wind up feeling isolated, guilty, and depressed. While doctors can support your treatment, a caring, willing support system will bolster you emotionally.

Support is also a practical matter. It can be a godsend to have someone to run and pick up your medication from the pharmacy when you're in the middle of a crushing migraine episode, or watch the kids when you're not up to it. In the most serious of circumstances, you might not be able to get to the doctor or the emergency room by yourself.

chapter 12

Emergency Care

Kim lived with migraine pain for years. With medication and other management strategies, she was beginning to get it under control. Every now and then she'd still have a real head banger, but as her treatment progressed, those became fewer and farther between. That's why it caught her by surprise when she awoke one night with what she described to us later as the worst headache of her life.

The headache was so powerful, she said it felt as if her head might explode. She was weak and dizzy. Her stomach churned, and she vomited several times. For the first time ever, she experienced a visual aura and light sensitivity. It was so frightening that she feared she might be having a stroke. Finally, when she could no longer tolerate the pain, she woke up her boyfriend and had him drive her to the emergency room or what doctors prefer to call the emergency department or ED.

As Kim discovered, reporting to the ED with a migraine is not always the greatest experience. Because she "only had a headache," the medical staff didn't seem to take her seriously. After all, it wasn't like she had a gunshot wound or was in the midst of a heart attack. After several agonizing hours of waiting on a stretcher in a noisy cubicle with fluorescent lights flickering above, a doctor finally did check her out. He was dismissive, though, and implied several times that he suspected her of exaggerating her symptoms in order to get narcotics. Once he was assured she wasn't a drug seeker, he still seemed tentative about how to handle her situation and reluctant to offer any treatment beyond a high-dose aspirin.

Many of our patients who've made a trip to the ED tell stories similar to Kim's. On the one hand, we can sympathize with these patients. Most people don't rush to the ED every time they experience some mild discomfort centered between their temples, so they don't appreciate being treated like a hypochondriac or desperate drug addict on the rare occasions when they do seek emergency care. On the other hand, ED staff don't usually have a lot of migraine-specific experience, so some may be reluctant or unsure of how to treat what can present as a fairly complex management issue. And from their point of view, drug-seeking ED patients complaining of various pains are not a rarity. Once they determine a headache isn't due to something life-threatening, like a stroke, they often find it easier to "treat 'em and street 'em."

Remember, Kim described her migraine as the *worst headache* she'd had in her life. A good rule of thumb is that an unusually severe or "different" headache is indeed a good reason to seek emergency evaluation. (For more guidance on when to seek emergency treatment see the "When to Worry" box on page 20.

However, while it's no sin to seek urgent care when necessary, it's never a good idea to use the ED for routine care. It's a very unproductive way to manage headaches. Your regular specialist has no control over what happens there, and since the ED doctor who sees you isn't likely to be familiar with your case, there's a good chance you could be subjected to a battery of unnecessary tests and scans that can be expensive or even carry health risks, such as exposure to radiation from computed tomography (CT) scans. Rushing to the hospital every time you have a migraine won't reward you with any friends among the ED staff, either.

Have a Plan

Someone who has recurring migraines should be prepared for emergency situations even when they don't end in a trip to the ED. We hope you'll never need to implement these plans, but if you do, you'll be grateful you thought ahead.

We recommend keeping an easily accessible list of important details about your headaches and medical history that you can hand over to an on-call doctor or attending ED physician. If you're in bad enough shape for urgent care, you may have trouble responding to questions clearly and accurately. Your list should include your diagnosis, treating physician's information, and emergency contacts, as well as a list of medications you currently take—both preventive and abortive—including dosages and frequency. Have your insurance information handy as well.

Think about what kind of support you'll need in times of emergency, such as someone to take you to the hospital and someone to cover responsibilities like child care, notifying your job, etc. Be sure to have discussions with each member of your support team so everyone is clear on his or her role. Keep their information in a handy place and consider placing your contacts on speed dial even if you know their numbers well—a whopping headache may cause you to temporarily forget basic information or make it difficult to dial the phone.

At your next doctor's visit, be sure to discuss what you can expect in terms of emergency care from your physician. Your doctor's practice may have an after-hours number to call for assistance as well as rules for when making such a call is acceptable. If not, ask your doctor what steps are recommended for when your medication fails to work and you are at a point where you can no longer stand the pain. Is there another practice you might see during off hours? Is there a particular preferred ED? Is there any circumstance where the doctor might agree to meet you at the ED? These are the sorts of answers you should have before you actually need them.

Included in this discussion with your doctor, ask about the possibility of "rescue medications." These are medications that should not be taken on a regular basis but can be considered as a last-ditch strategy in lieu of, or before, taking that trip to the ED.

Rescue medications should only be taken in the event that every other medication, treatment, and strategy fails for a particular migraine episode, and you must have relief. Many rescue drugs are stronger than routine medications and carry a risk of more serious side effects or the possibility of addiction. Long-term use of such drugs is rare and only considered in specialty care and special cases. Other rescue medications are typical abortive drugs that come in a suppository, nasal spray, or injectable form for faster delivery or because they're tolerated better than drugs that must be swallowed.

You and your doctor can make the decision whether rescue medications are preferable to the trip to the ED or whether you should accept a rescue medication as part of emergency treatment. But rescue medications should *never* be the first line of treatment. If you find yourself using them on a regular basis, you and your doctor must work together to make changes in routine treatment.

Emergency-care strategies work best when everyone involved is on the same page; most importantly, you and your doctor must be on the same page. We believe the doctor's role is to offer advice about managing the overall pattern of your headaches, and the patient's role is to carry out and test different management strategies for acute migraine episodes. Of course, for times when you truly need your doctor's immediate advice, most doctors will do their best to help. However, it's important to keep things in perspective: No doctor can be there to treat each and every individual headache or offer immediate advice about changes in treatment strategy. Instead, you might want to adopt an attitude that you are "field testing" various treatment strategies, then returning to your doctor with information about what worked and what didn't. Then the two of you together can formulate an updated, altered treatment strategy that you can take charge of carrying out.

chapter 13

Final Thoughts

We want to be completely honest with you: We don't always get a patient's treatment right on the first try—or multiple tries—so there can be some trial and error to migraine treatment. It's also part of our full disclosure that current treatments for migraines are far from perfect. If we could wave a wand over your forehead and wish for a magic cure, we would—and we're sure your doctor would do the same. But unfortunately, that's not how medicine works.

Does that mean you should feel discouraged and immediately give up? Absolutely not. You should look upon these facts as good news. If one medication doesn't work, it's possible that another one will. Or that it will work in combination with other drugs or nondrug treatments—or it may work for you in the future. Changing one lifestyle habit may not make that much of a difference but tweaking another one may make all the difference in the frequency and severity of your headaches. Or if acupuncture turns out to be a bust, biofeedback may turn out to be your ticket to a headache-free life.

We understand and sympathize with how easy it is to get discouraged when a round of migraine treatment doesn't solve your problems. You may feel like giving up. But we urge you to hang in there and keep trying. Throughout our years of treating those who suffer from migraines, we've found we've been able to improve the lives of the vast majority of our patients. In many cases, we've been able to resolve their headache issues almost entirely.

But rarely does this happen with a wave of a wand or as quickly as a patient would like. We often remind our patients that they've likely been suffering with migraines for years, so they should not expect the solutions to come overnight. They will be rewarded if they hang in with their treatment and work with their medical team to come up with the combination of therapies and treatments that are right for their personal circumstances.

While we believe that the information in this book can help most people who suffer from migraines get on the right track, we have seen a few patients who don't respond very well to any sort of treatment over a long period of time. Although we tend to discourage medication- and doctor-hopping, we do encourage you to keep trying new things even if everything has failed thus far. It may feel like you've tried everything, but there's still that throbbing pain in the temple that comes with alarming frequency. In some patients whose severe headaches do not respond to aggressive outpatient treatment, hospitalization in a specialty headache unit may be helpful. There are only a handful of such programs in the United States, however, so orchestrating and getting insurance approval for such therapy can be a challenge.

Don't give up hope! There are new information, medications, procedures, and therapies coming out for migraines all the time. We encourage you to keep trying. And we hope your medical and support team continue to work with you until you make peace with migraine pain once and for all.

chapter 14

Resources

Here, we've provided a list of further reading and resources should you wish to pursue information beyond what we've included in this book. This is by no means an exhaustive list of materials, Web sites, and organizations aimed at helping people who suffer from migraines. However, we're satisfied that it represents a wide scope of credible and high-quality resources. Although we don't necessarily endorse every notion put forth by the various organizations and resources listed, we are satisfied that they all offer high-quality information that can be beneficial for understanding and managing migraines. We recommend you also check state and local listings for additional resources in your area.

Migraine and Headache

Alliance for Headache Disorders Advocacy

The AHDA is a consortium of nonprofit organizations with an interest in headache disorders. It is dedicated to advocacy efforts "that can result in better treatment for all headache disorder patients." The AHDA sponsors an annual "Headache on the Hill" visit to congressional representatives to advocate for better research funding for headache disorders. It also provides a mechanism for headache patients and others to easily contact their congressional representatives via e-mail when legislative matters relating to headache are considered by Congress.

http://www.allianceforheadacheadvocacy.org/who_is.htm

American Council for Headache Education (ACHE) and the American Headache Society

19 Mantua Rd.
Mt. Royal, NJ 08061
Phone: (856) 423-0258
Toll-free: (800) 255-2243
Fax: (856) 423-0082

E-mail: achehq@talley.com
http://www.achenet.org/

ACHE is the education arm of the American Headache Society (AHS). AHS is a professional society of health-care providers dedicated to the study and treatment of headache and face pain. ACHE exists primarily as an educational resource for physicians, health-care providers, and patients who seek resources and educational information on headaches. The Web site provides information about a number of headache topics, including information in Spanish. These informational leaflets and several headache diaries are available for download and printing.

American Migraine Foundation

The AMF is a charitable foundation administered by the American Headache Society. Its goal is to raise money "to support innovative research that will lead to improvement in the lives of those who suffer from migraine and other disabling headaches."

http://www.americanmigrainefoundation.org

Help for Headaches and Migraine

This is a useful Web site created and maintained by Teri Robert, a person with migraines who has become a headache educator and an activist for improved funding for migraine research and treatment.

Teri Robert
P.O. Box 1726
Parkersburg, WV 26102-1726
E-mail: teri@helpforheadaches.com
http://www.helpforheadaches.com/

International Headache Foundation

The International Headache Society is an international professional organization for those who treat headache problems. The society publishes the criteria used to diagnose and classify headaches, and provides money for fellowship training in headache.

www.ihs-headache.org/frame_non_members.asp

National Headache Foundation

428 West Saint James Place
2nd Floor
Chicago, IL 60614-2750
Toll-free: (800) 643-5552
E-mail: info@headaches.org
http://www.headaches.org/

The world's largest voluntary organization for the support of headache sufferers. The organization provides people-to-people support to those who struggle with frequent and extreme headaches and gives health-care providers and their patients access to resources.

National Institute of Neurological Disorders and Stroke

P.O. Box 5801
Bethesda, MD 20824
Toll-Free: (800) 352-9424
http://www.ninds.nih.gov/

The mission of the National Institute of Neurological Disorders and Stroke is to reduce the burden of neurological disease—a burden borne by every age group, by every segment of society, by people all over the world.

Lifestyle Resources

American Academy of Sleep Medicine

2510 North Frontage Road
Darien, IL 60561
Phone: (708) 492-0930
Fax: (630) 737-9790
www.aasmnet.org
www.sleepeducation.com

The American Academy of Sleep Medicine (AASM) is the only professional society dedicated exclusively to the medical subspecialty of sleep medicine. As the leading voice in the field of sleep medicine, the AASM sets standards and promotes excellence in health care, education, and research.

National Sleep Foundation

1522 K Street, NW, Suite 500
Washington, DC 20005
Phone: (202) 347-3471
Fax: (202) 347-3472
E-mail: nsf@sleepfoundation.org
www.sleepfoundation.org

Alerting the public, health-care providers, and policymakers to the life-and-death importance of adequate sleep is central to the mission of NSF. NSF is dedicated to improving the quality of life for Americans who suffer from sleep problems and disorders. This means helping the public better understand the importance of sleep and the benefits of good sleep habits, and recognizing the signs of sleep problems so that they can be properly diagnosed and treated.

American Council on Exercise (ACE)

4851 Paramount Drive
San Diego, CA 92123
Phone: (858) 576-6500
Toll-free: (888) 825-3636
Fax: (858) 576-6564
E-mail: resource@acefitness.org
www.acefitness.org

This organization serves as America's Authority on Fitness® by equipping fitness professionals and consumers with credible information, resources, research, and tools on safe and effective exercise and fitness products, programs, and trends. It connects consumers with certified professionals through outreach, online tools, and social networking and partners with consumers to empower them to reach their health and fitness goals.

American College of Sports Medicine (ACSM)

P.O. Box 1440
Indianapolis, IN 46206-1440
Phone: (317) 637-9200
Fax: (317) 634-7817
www.acsm.org

The American College of Sports Medicine promotes and integrates scientific research, education, and practical applications of sports medicine and exercise science to maintain and enhance physical performance, fitness, health, and quality of life.

American Heart Association

7272 Greenville Ave.
Dallas, TX 75231
Phone: (800) AHA-USA-1
www.heart.org

The mission of this organization is to build healthier lives free of cardiovascular diseases and stroke.

American Dietetic Association

120 South Riverside Plaza, Suite 2000
Chicago, IL 60606-6995
Phone: (312) 899-0040
Toll-free: (800) 877-1600
www.eatright.org

The American Dietetic Association is the world's largest organization of food and nutrition professionals. ADA is committed to improving the nation's health and advancing the profession of dietetics through research, education, and advocacy.

Complementary and Alternative Medicine (CAM)

National Center for Complementary and Alternative Medicine (NCCAM)

National Institutes of Health
P.O. Box 7923
Gaithersburg, MD 20898
Toll-free: (888) 644-6226
Fax: (866) 464-3616

TTY: (866) 464-3615
http://nccam.nih.gov/

Part of the National Institutes of Health, this government agency offers a wealth of publications on a variety of health problems. It also sponsors valuable research on alternative and complementary medicine.

Association for Applied Psychophysiology and Biofeedback

10200 W. 44th Ave, Suite 304
Wheat Ridge, CO 80033-2840
Toll-free: (800) 477-8892
http://www.aapb.org/

AAPB's mission is to advance the development, dissemination, and utilization of knowledge about applied psychophysiology and biofeedback to improve health and the quality of life through research, education, and practice.

American Massage Therapy Association

500 Davis St., Suite 900
Evanston, IL 60201

Toll-free: (877) 905-2700
www.amtamassage.org

The professional association for massage therapists offers a therapist locator service on its Web site.

American Physical Therapy Association

1111 N. Fairfax St.
Alexandria, VA 22314
Toll-free: (800) 999-2782
www.apta.org

This national professional organization for physical therapists provides information on preventing and treating neck pain and on maintaining good posture throughout life.

Biofeedback Certification Institute of America

10200 W. 44th Ave., Suite 310
Wheat Ridge, CO 80033
Toll-free: (866) 908-8713
www.bcia.org

This organization certifies practitioners in biofeedback. Its Web site offers general information on biofeedback and a search engine to find practitioners with various specialties, including physical therapy, neuromuscular rehabilitation, and pain.

National Certification Commission for Acupuncture and Oriental Medicine

76 S. Laura St., Suite 1290
Jacksonville, FL 32202
Phone: (904) 598-1005
www.nccaom.org

This organization establishes, assesses, and promotes recognized standards of competence and safety in acupuncture and Oriental medicine for the protection and benefit of the public.

The National Resource Center for Domestic Violence

3605 Vartan Way
Harrisburg, PA 17110
Phone: (800) 537-2238 ext. 5
Fax: 717-545-9456
Toll-free: (800) 799-7233 or (800) 787-3224.
http://www.nrcdv.org/tips.php

Because the incidence of migraine is sometimes linked to past abuse or domestic violence, we believe it is useful to provide information and resources about domestic violence and its prevention. The Web site includes specific tips and strategies for those who are experiencing domestic violence and provides information about how to get help.

On the Internet

Center for Mindfulness in Medicine, Health Care and Society

University of Massachusetts Medical School
Worcester, MA
http://www.umassmed.edu/content.aspx?id=41252

Provides information on mindfulness and offers mindfulness-based stress-reduction programs. Founded by Jon Kabat-Zinn, Ph.D.—author of numerous scientific papers on the clinical applications of mindfulness; instructor in mindfulness and MBSR; and author of several books for lay audiences, including *Full Catastrophe Living: Using the Wisdom of Your Body and Mind to Face Stress* and *Wherever You Go, There You Are: Mindfulness Meditation in*

Everyday Life. Kabat-Zinn's mindfulness meditation books, CDs, and tapes may be ordered at http://www.mindful nesscds/index.html.

Benson-Henry Institute for Mind-Body Medicine

Massachusetts General Hospital
Boston, MA
http://www.massgeneral.org/bhi/default.aspx

Under the direction of Harvard Medical School's Dr. Herbert Benson, who pioneered the "relaxation response," the Benson-Henry Institute works to advance the study and practice of mind-body medicine. On the Benson-Henry Web site, you can find an overview of mind-body medicine, as well as information and instructions in mindfulness practice, stress management, and eliciting the relaxation response. Books, CDs, and tapes are available through the Web site.

"Healthy Sleep"

http://healthysleep.med.harvard.edu

Created by Harvard Medical School's Division of Sleep Medicine and the WGBH Educational Foundation, this

Web site discusses the science of sleep and ways to get the sleep you need.

Harvard Health Publications Special Health Reports

Stress Management: Approaches for Preventing and Reducing Stress (2008) covers the stress response, causes of stress, and strategies for preventing or reducing stress. Includes relaxation and mindfulness techniques.

Understanding Depression (2008) focuses on depression and its treatment. Offers information on mindfulness and instructions for performing mindfulness exercises.

Positive Psychology: Harnessing the Power of Happiness, Personal Strength, and Mindfulness (2009); a guide to the concept of positive psychology, which studies the relationship between positive emotions and greater health and well-being. Includes a section on mindfulness techniques.

Center for Mindfulness in Medicine, Health Care, and Society

55 Lake Ave. N.
Worcester, MA 01655
Phone: (508) 856-2656
www.umassmed.edu/cfm

Founded by Jon Kabat-Zinn, author of *Full Catastrophe Living*, the center offers information and programs on stress reduction. Its clinical treatment program is affiliated with the University of Massachusetts Medical School.

Additional Reading

Harvard Medical School Guide to Lowering Your Blood Pressure
Aggie Casey, M.S., R.N., and Herbert Benson, M.D.
(McGraw-Hill, 2005, 256 pages)

Harvard Medical School experts present an innovative, proven plan to lower your blood pressure. In addition to offering nutrition and exercise advice, the book describes techniques that can help you manage your stress levels.

Living Well with Migraine Disease and Headaches: What Your Doctor Doesn't Tell You . . . That You Need to Know
Teri Robert
(HarperCollins, 2005, 301 pages)

This is a comprehensive review of migraine and other chronic headaches, written by migraine sufferer, patient advocate, and educator Teri Robert. One of our favorites, this book provides information from the patient's point of view about navigating life with chronic headaches.

Mind Your Heart: A Mind/Body Approach to Stress Management, Exercise, and Nutrition for Heart Health
Aggie Casey, M.S., R.N., and Herbert Benson, M.D., with Ann MacDonald
(Free Press, 2004, 352 pages)

Offers a balanced and holistic approach to heart health that combines lifestyle changes with cutting-edge medical procedures. Discusses the importance of risk factors such as depression, anger and hostility, decreased social support, physical inactivity, and poor nutrition, and outlines self-care strategies to combat these problems.

The Relaxation Response (updated and expanded edition)
Herbert Benson, M.D., with Miriam Z. Klipper
(Avon Books, 2000, 240 pages)

A groundbreaking book that revealed the health benefits of stress-management techniques. This revised classic describes the therapeutic effects of the relaxation response and teaches a variety of methods to elicit it.

Self-Nurture: Learning to Care for Yourself as Effectively as You Care for Everyone Else
Alice D. Domar, Ph.D., and Henry Dreher
(Penguin Books, 2001, 320 pages)

Written for women, this book offers a prescription for enrichment and self-nurture techniques intended to revitalize your life and reconnect your body to your mind.

"Conquering Insomnia"
www.cbtforinsomnia.com

This cognitive behavioral-therapy program, developed by Dr. Gregg Jacobs at Harvard Medical School and the University of Massachusetts Medical Center, can be purchased as an online program or in CD format ($29.95).

At-a-Glance Resources and References

Health History Questionnaire

Here is the form we ask patients to fill out and bring along with them to their first visit. We find that going through the process of completing this form at home gives patients a chance to think carefully about the history of their headaches (which sometimes is long and complicated). It also gives them a chance to seek more information from family members or other doctors about things they may have forgotten.

You may find it useful to fill out this form and bring it to your initial visit with a specialist. Many specialists use a similar form or will at least ask you similar questions to those listed on this questionnaire.

MIDAS (Migraine Disability Assessment) Questionnaire

This is another typical form that many doctors use to assess the degree of migraine disability you experience. The MIDAS questionnaire was put together to help you measure the impact your headaches have on your life. The information on this questionnaire is also helpful for your primary-care provider to determine the level of pain and disability caused by your headaches and to find the best treatment for you.

Instructions

Please answer the following questions about ALL of the headaches you have had over the last three months. Select

HEALTH HISTORY QUESTIONNAIRE

Name *(Last, First, M.I.)*: ☐ M ☐ F | **Birth date:**

Marital status: ☐ Single ☐ Partnered ☐ Married ☐ Separated ☐ Divorced ☐ Widowed

Referring doctor:

Are you RIGHT, LEFT handed or ambidextrous?

Highest Level of Education:

List any medical problems that other doctors have diagnosed

Surgeries

Year	Reason	Hospital

Other hospitalizations

Year	Reason	Hospital

List your prescribed drugs and over-the-counter drugs, such as vitamins and inhalers

Name the Drug	Strength	Frequency Taken

Allergies or bad reactions to medications

Name the Drug	Reaction You Had

HEALTH HABITS AND PERSONAL SAFETY

ALL QUESTIONS CONTAINED IN THIS QUESTIONNAIRE ARE OPTIONAL AND WILL BE KEPT STRICTLY CONFIDENTIAL.					
Exercise	☐ Sedentary (No exercise)				
	☐ Mild exercise (i.e., climb stairs, walk 3 blocks, golf)				
	☐ Occasional vigorous exercise (i.e., work or recreation, less than 4x/week for 30 min.)				
	☐ Regular vigorous exercise (i.e., work or recreation 4x/week for 30 minutes)				
Diet	Are you dieting?			☐ Yes	☐ No
	# of meals you eat in an average day?				
	Rank salt intake	☐ High	☐ Med	☐ Low	
	Rank fat intake	☐ High	☐ Med	☐ Low	
Caffeine	☐ None	☐ Coffee	☐ Tea	☐ Cola	
	# of cups/cans per day?				
Alcohol	Do you drink alcohol?			☐ Yes	☐ No
	If yes, what kind?				

	How many drinks per week?		
	Are you concerned about the amount you drink?	☐ Yes	☐ No
	Have you considered stopping?	☐ Yes	☐ No
	Have you ever experienced blackouts?	☐ Yes	☐ No
	Are you prone to "binge" drinking?	☐ Yes	☐ No
Tobacco	Do you use tobacco?	☐ Yes	☐ No
	☐ Cigarettes—pks./day		
	☐ # of years	☐ Or year quit	
Drugs	Do you currently use recreational or street drugs?	☐ Yes	☐ No
Sex	Are you sexually active?	☐ Yes	☐ No
	If yes, are you trying for a pregnancy?	☐ Yes	☐ No
	If not trying for a pregnancy list contraceptive or barrier method used:		
Personal Safety	Do you live alone?	☐ Yes	☐ No
	Do you have frequent falls?	☐ Yes	☐ No
	Do you have vision or hearing loss?	☐ Yes	☐ No

FAMILY HEALTH HISTORY

	AGE	SIGNIFICANT HEALTH PROBLEMS		AGE
Father			**Children**	☐ M ☐ F
Mother				☐ M ☐ F
Sibling	☐ M ☐ F			☐ M ☐ F
	☐ M ☐ F			☐ M ☐ F
	☐ M ☐ F		**Grandmother** *Maternal*	
	☐ M ☐ F		**Grandfather** *Maternal*	
	☐ M ☐ F		**Grandmother** *Paternal*	
	☐ M ☐ F		**Grandfather** *Paternal*	

MENTAL HEALTH

Question	Yes	No
Is stress a major problem for you?	☐ Yes	☐ No
Do you feel depressed?	☐ Yes	☐ No
Do you have problems with eating or your appetite?	☐ Yes	☐ No
Have you ever attempted suicide or seriously thought about hurting yourself?	☐ Yes	☐ No
Do you have trouble sleeping?	☐ Yes	☐ No
Have you ever been to a counselor?	☐ Yes	☐ No

************ FOR WOMEN ONLY *************** FOR WOMEN ONLY ***************

Question	Yes	No
Age at onset of menstruation:		
Date of last menstruation:		
Period every ________ days		
Number of pregnancies ________ Number of live births ________		
Are you pregnant or breastfeeding?	☐ Yes	☐ No
Have you had a hysterectomy?	☐ Yes	☐ No
Any problems with control of urination?	☐ Yes	☐ No
Any hot flashes or sweating at night?	☐ Yes	☐ No
Do you have menstrual tension, pain, bloating, irritability, or other symptoms at or around time of period?	☐ Yes	☐ No

************ FOR MEN ONLY **************** FOR MEN ONLY *******************

Do you usually get up to urinate during the night?	☐ Yes	☐ No
If yes, # of times ________		
Do you have any problems emptying your bladder completely?	☐ Yes	☐ No
Any difficulty with erection or ejaculation?	☐ Yes	☐ No

OTHER PROBLEMS

Check and circle if you have, or have had, any symptoms in the following areas to a significant degree and briefly explain below.

☐ Skin: Mole, rash, itching, dryness	☐ Chest/Heart: Palpitations, pain	**Recent changes in:**
☐ Head/Neck/Throat: Sinus problems, sore throat, lumps	☐ Back: Pain, stiffness	☐ Weight
☐ Ears: Ear pain, ringing, hearing loss	☐ Intestinal	☐ Energy level
☐ Speech or swallowing difficulty	☐ Bladder/bowel: Incontinence, constipation	☐ Ability to sleep
☐ Nose: Pain, stuffy, discharge	☐ Circulation: Cold extremities, color change	☐ Other pain/discomfort:
☐ Lungs: Cough, shortness of breath	☐ Fevers/chills/sweats	☐
☐ Joint aches, pains or swelling	☐	☐
☐	☐	☐

your answer in the box next to each question. Select zero if you did not have the activity in the last three months.

1. On how many days in the last three months did you miss work or school because of your headaches?
2. How many days in the last three months was your productivity at work or school reduced by half or more because of your headaches? (Do not include days you counted in question 1 where you missed work or school.)
3. On how many days in the last three months did you not do household work (such as housework, home repairs and maintenance, shopping, caring for children and relatives) because of your headaches?
4. How many days in the last three months was your productivity in household work reduced by half or more because of your headaches? (Do not include days you counted in question 3 where you did not do household work.)
5. On how many days in the last three months did you miss family, social, or leisure activities because of your headaches?

Total (Questions 1–5)

On how many days in the last three months did you have a headache? (If a headache lasted more than one day, count each day.)

On a scale of 0–10, on average how painful were these headaches? (where 0 = no pain at all, and 10 = pain as bad as it can be.)

MIDAS Grade	Definition	MIDAS Score
I	Little or no disability	0–5
II	Mild disability	6–10
III	Moderate disability	11–20
IV	Severe disability	21+

Migraine Trigger Checklist

Although as we explain in chapter 3, we don't think it's wise to spend too much time thinking about your migraine triggers, especially those over which you have little or no control, it can be useful at the outset of treatment to try to identify things that influence the chance you will get a headache. However, it pays to keep in mind that triggers are often multifactorial and sometimes quite weak—so while it may seem that a particular thing or circumstance is a culprit, the reality is often more complicated than that.

_______ Aged cheeses

_______ Alcohol (red wine, beer, whiskey, champagne)

_______ Caffeine (excess intake or withdrawal)

_______ Chocolate

_______ Citrus fruits

_______ Cured meats

_______ Dehydration

_______ Depression

_______ Diet (skipping meals or fasting)

_______ Dried fish

_______ Dried fruits

_______ Exercise (excessive)

_______ Eyestrain or other visual triggers

_______ Fatigue (extreme)

_______ Food additives (nitrites, nitrates, MSG)

_______ Lights (bright or flickering; sunlight)

_______ Lunch meats

_______ Menstrual periods

_______ Medications

_______ MSG

_______ Noise (excessive)

_______ NutraSweet®

_______ Nuts

_______ Odors

_______ Onions

_______ Salty foods

_______ Sleep (too much, too little, other changes)

_______ Skipped meals

_______ Stress

_______ Television or movie viewing

_______ Weather (changing conditions)

_______ Wine (red)

_______ Others

Possible triggers:

Migraine 1:

Migraine 2:

Migraine 3:

Migraine 4:

Prodrome Symptom Checklist

It's often more effective to treat a migraine either before or as close to the onset as possible. This list includes many of the symptoms and warning signs that a migraine is on its way or in its early stages. You may find it useful to refer to this checklist to help you learn to recognize your migraines before they become full-blown. Share this with your doctor. A specialist can work with you to see if catching and responding to headaches early improves the results you get from treatment.

Fatigue	Blurry vision
Nausea, stomach upset	Visual aura
Vomiting	Nervousness
Sinus pressure	Hunger
Sensitivity to smells	Food craving
Moodiness	Dizzy spells
Light-headedness	Noise sensitivity
Light sensitivity	Achy muscles
Thirst	Skin sensitivity
Stomach pain	Stiff or achy neck
Nasal congestion	Teary eyes
Irritability	Anxiety
Difficulty concentrating	Yawning
Flu-like symptoms	Other

What symptoms did you experience?

Migraine 1:

Migraine 2:

Migraine 3:

Migraine 4:

Simple Headache Diary

This diary form is fairly self-explanatory. Simply fill in the chart each time you have a headache. If you have more than three episodes in a time period, you will need to reproduce this sheet multiple times.

	First episode	Second episode	Third episode
Date/day of the week of headache			
Time of onset			
Time of resolution			
Warning signs			
Location(s) of the pain			
Type of pain (e.g. sharp, dull, steady, throb)			
Maximum intensity of the pain*			
Additional symptoms			
Activities/circumstances at time of onset			
Time of most recent meal prior to onset			

	First episode	Second episode	Third episode
Food/drink most recently consumed prior to onset			
Medication(s) taken for headache			
Response to medication(s)			
Other action(s) taken for relief			
Response to action(s)			
Last menstrual period**			
Medication(s) currently taken for other condition(s)			
*on a scale from 1 to 10, with 1 being very mild pain and 10 being the worst pain possible **beginning date and ending date			
Note: Permission is granted to reproduce this page of the report for individual use.			

Migraine Team Checklist

A list of important contacts

	Name	Address	Phone	E-mail	Fax
Migraine Specialist					
Primary-Care Doctor or Nurse-Practitioner					
Pharmacy					
Emergency Clinic					
Support team #1					
Support team #2					
Support team #3					

Migraine Medication Checklist

	Dosage	Frequency	Time of Day Taken	Notes
Preventive Medication #1				
Preventive Medication #2				
Abortive Medication #1				
Abortive Medication #2				
Antinausea Medication				
Other Medication				
Other Medication				
Supplements, vitamins, or herbs				
Other Treatment				
Other Treatment				

Reference List of Preventive Medications		
Preventive Medications	Dose (mg)	Duration (days, weeks, etc.)
Atenolol (Tenormin®)		
Metoprolol (Toprol XL®)		
Nadolol (Corgard®)		
Propranolol (Inderal®)		
Tinolol (Blocadren®)		
Verapamil (Calan® and others)		
Amitriptyline (Elavil®)		
Nortriptyline (Pamelor®)		
Imipramine (Tofranil® and others)		
Lisinopril (Vasotec®)		
Candesartan (Atacand®)		
Valproate (Depakote®, Depakote® ER, etc.)		
Gabapentin (Neurontin®)		
Pregabalin (Lyrica®)		
Topiramate (Topamax®)		
Indomethacin (Indocin®)		
Onabotulinum Toxin A (Botox® injections)		
Nerve Blocks/ Trigger-point injections		

Reference List of Abortive Medications		
Prescription Abortive Medications used per month	Dose/Route (for example, "by mouth")	Typical amount
Ibuprofen (Motrin®)		
Ketoprofen (Orudis®)		
Naproxen (Naprosyn®)		
Naratriptan (Amerge®)		
Almotriptan (Axert®)		
Frovatriptan (Frova®)		
Sumatriptan (Imitrex®)		
Rizatriptan (Maxalt®)		
Eletriptan (Relpax®)		
Zolmitriptan (Zomig®)		
Dihydroergotamine (D.H.E. 45®, Migranal®)		
Ergotamine tartrate/ caffeine (Cafergot®)		
Promethazine (Phenergan®)		
Prochlorperazine (Compazine®)		
Metoclopramide (Reglan®)		

Butalbital/caffeine/ ASA or acetaminophen		
(Fioricet®, Fiorinal®, Esgic®)		
Butalbital/Acetaminophen (Phrenilin®)		
Opioids (codeine, Percocet®, Vicodin®, Oxycontin®, fentanyl, Stadol®, etc.)		
Steroids (Medrol®, decadron, prednisone)		

Over-the-counter/ supplements	Dose/# tablets	Typical amount used per month
Excedrin®/Excedrin® Migraine/Excedrin® Tension, Anacin®, etc.		
Tylenol®/Tylenol® Sinus, etc.		
Decongestants		
Motrin®/Motrin® Migraine, etc.		
Aspirin		
Advil®		
Aleve®		
Magnesium		
MigreLief®		
Vitamin B_2		
Petadolex® (butterbur)		
Coenzyme Q10		
Bufferin®		
Melatonin		
Feverfew		

Acknowledgments

We'd like to acknowledge the following people for helping make this book become a reality:

Julie Silver, MD, chief editor in books at Harvard Health Publications, who conceived the idea for this project and assembled the author team. We thank you for your tireless patience and advocacy.

Tony Komaroff, MD, editor in chief of Harvard Health Publications. We appreciate your passion for bringing to the public medical information that is practical, accessible, and accurate.

Linda Konner, our literary agent. Your ability to shape a project and bring all parties to the table is unparalleled.

Meredith Mennitt, our wonderful St. Martin's Press

editor who diplomatically helped guide us through the book writing process and made our pages all the better for it.

Finally, we'd like to thank our wonderful families for taking up the slack and giving us the time and support we needed to do our day jobs and write this book.

Index